Student Nurse Practitioner Clinical Notebook

By
Nachole Johnson, FNP-BC

ISBN-13: 978-1548958282
ISBN-10: 154895828X
Printed in the United States of America
10 9 8 7 6 5 4 3 2 1

Why I Wrote This Book

As a nurse who has "nursed" on many levels - CNA, LPN, RN, BSN and MSN, I realize how important it is to be organized for the patients you are caring for. I never really had a good process for documenting my clinical experiences while I attended school. I hated printing out clinical sheets and carrying around tons of loose paperwork to each clinical rotation. The worse part was to go through all this paperwork at the end of the semester to log my time or find the notes on the interesting pediatric patient I had two months prior. I tried carrying around a simple notebook at one point, but it still lacked the organization I needed for clinicals.

Being organized for clinicals is key to having a great clinical experience. By keeping all of your clinical notes in one book, you have a reference to look back on at the end of your semester to learn from your patient encounters in clinicals. You will also have a handy reference for when you need to log each patient into your clinical tracking system to document all your patient experiences and hours.

The notebook includes daily History & Physical sheets for you to document pertinent patient information. The two- page History & Physical sheets are formatted to lie side-by-side for easy note taking and there are plenty of spaces within the template to write additional notes about your clinical day.

My hope is that this clinical notebook becomes a valuable part of your toolkit while in school to make one part of your nurse practitioner school experience less stressful.

Enjoy!

- *Nachole*

Clinical Rotation_____   Date: _____

Chief Complaint:
_____

History of Present Illness:
_____
_____
_____
_____
_____

Review of Systems:

	Yes	No		Yes	No		Yes	No		Yes	No
General: fatigue	[]	[]	CV: chest pain	[]	[]	Bloody stool	[]	[]	Polydypsia	[]	[]
Weight loss	[]	[]	Edema	[]	[]	GU: dysuria	[]	[]	Polyphagia	[]	[]
Fever	[]	[]	PND	[]	[]	Frequency	[]	[]	Polyphagia	[]	[]
Chills	[]	[]	Orthopnea	[]	[]	Hematuria	[]	[]	Temp int	[]	[]
Night sweats	[]	[]	Palpitations	[]	[]	Discharge	[]	[]	Derm: rash	[]	[]
Eye: vision change	[]	[]	Claudication	[]	[]	Flank pain	[]	[]	Pruritis	[]	[]
Pain	[]	[]	Resp: cough	[]	[]	MS: arthralgia	[]	[]	Neuro: weakness	[]	[]
Redness	[]	[]	SOB	[]	[]	Arthritis	[]	[]	Seizures	[]	[]
ENT: headaches	[]	[]	Wheezing	[]	[]	Joint swelling	[]	[]	Parasthesias	[]	[]
Hoarseness	[]	[]	Hemoptysis	[]	[]	Myalgias	[]	[]	Tremors	[]	[]
Sore throat	[]	[]	GI: abd pain	[]	[]	Back pain	[]	[]	Syncope	[]	[]
Epistaxis	[]	[]	BM changes	[]	[]	Heme: bleeding	[]	[]	Psych: anxiety	[]	[]
Sinus Sx	[]	[]	N/V	[]	[]	Bruising	[]	[]	Depression	[]	[]
Hearing loss	[]	[]	Diarrhea	[]	[]	Lymph: swelling	[]	[]	Hallucinations	[]	[]
Tinnitus	[]	[]	Heartburn	[]	[]	Endo: polyuria	[]	[]	All/Imm: hayfever	[]	[]
									Runny nose	[]	[]

Other ROS: _____

Past Medical History:
_____
_____
_____
_____
_____
_____
_____

Past Surgical History:
_____
_____
_____

Family History:
_____
_____

[] All other ROS reviewed and were NEGATIVE

Social History:
_____

Cigs: [] No Yes [] → Pack yrs _____
ETOH [] No Yes [] → Amount? _____
Illicits [] No Yes [] → Type?   _____
Allergies: [] NKDA _____
Medications:
_____
_____
_____
_____
_____
_____
_____

Physical Exam T _____ BP _____ HR _____ Wt _____(lbs) Ht _____(in) BMI _____		
Eyes [] nl conjunctiva & lids	**ENT** External [] no scars, lesions, masses	**Neck** External [] no tracheal deviation
Pupils [] equal, round, & reactive	Otoscopic [] nl canals, TM	Palpation [] no masses
Fundus [] nl discs and vessels	Hearing [] nl hearing	Thyroid [] no enlargement
Vision [] acuity & gross fields intact	Oropharynx [] nl teeth, tongue, pharynx	Abnormals:
Abnormals:	Abnormals:	
GI Palpation [] no masses or tenderness [] no hep/splenomegaly	**Resp** Effort [] nl w/o retractions	**Skin** [] no rashes, or lesions
Ausculation [] nl bowel sounds	Percussion [] no dullness	Chest [] nl breast, no d/c
Percussion [] no dullness	Palpation [] no fremitus	Lymph nodes [] no axillary, inguinal, cervical or submandibular LAD
Anus/rectum [] no abnormality or masses [] heme negative stool	Ausculation [] CTA w/o W, R, or R	GU [] nl male/female exam
Abnormals:	Abnormals:	Psych [] nl cognition
CV Palpation [] PMI nondisplaced	**Neuro** Orientation [] AAO x 3	Abnormals:
Auscultation [] no murmur, gallop, or rub	Cranial nerves [] CN II-XII intact	
Carotids [] nl intensity w/o bruit	Sensory [] nl sensation	
JVD [] no jugulovenous distention	Reflexes [] 2+ & symmetrical	
Pulses [] 2+/= femoral & pedal pulses	Abnormals:	
Edema [] no pedal edema		
Abnormals		

Musculoskeletal	Inspection	ROM	Strength	Tone (✓ if normal)	Abnormals:	**Other:**
Upper extremity	[]	[]	[]	[]		
Lower extremity	[]	[]	[]	[]		
Gait	[] nl gait and FROM					

Labs:

Assessment & Plan:

_____
_____
_____
_____
_____
_____
_____
_____
_____
_____

Clinical Rotation_____   Date: _____

Chief Complaint:

_____

History of Present Illness:

_____
_____
_____
_____
_____

Review of Systems:

	Yes	No		Yes	No		Yes	No		Yes	No
General: fatigue	[]	[]	CV: chest pain	[]	[]	Bloody stool	[]	[]	Polydypsia	[]	[]
Weight loss	[]	[]	Edema	[]	[]	GU: dysuria	[]	[]	Polyphagia	[]	[]
Fever	[]	[]	PND	[]	[]	Frequency	[]	[]	Polyphagia	[]	[]
Chills	[]	[]	Orthopnea	[]	[]	Hematuria	[]	[]	Temp int	[]	[]
Night sweats	[]	[]	Palpitations	[]	[]	Discharge	[]	[]	Derm: rash	[]	[]
Eye: vision change	[]	[]	Claudication	[]	[]	Flank pain	[]	[]	Pruritis	[]	[]
Pain	[]	[]	Resp: cough	[]	[]	MS: arthralgia	[]	[]	Neuro: weakness	[]	[]
Redness	[]	[]	SOB	[]	[]	Arthritis	[]	[]	Seizures	[]	[]
ENT: headaches	[]	[]	Wheezing	[]	[]	Joint swelling	[]	[]	Parasthesias	[]	[]
Hoarseness	[]	[]	Hemoptysis	[]	[]	Myalgias	[]	[]	Tremors	[]	[]
Sore throat	[]	[]	GI: abd pain	[]	[]	Back pain	[]	[]	Syncope	[]	[]
Epistaxis	[]	[]	BM changes	[]	[]	Heme: bleeding	[]	[]	Psych: anxiety	[]	[]
Sinus Sx	[]	[]	N/V	[]	[]	Bruising	[]	[]	Depression	[]	[]
Hearing loss	[]	[]	Diarrhea	[]	[]	Lymph: swelling	[]	[]	Hallucinations	[]	[]
Tinnitus	[]	[]	Heartburn	[]	[]	Endo: polyuria	[]	[]	All/Imm: hayfever	[]	[]
									Runny nose	[]	[]

Other ROS: _____

Past Medical History:

_____
_____
_____
_____
_____
_____
_____

Past Surgical History:

_____
_____
_____
_____

Family History:

_____
_____

[] All other ROS reviewed and were NEGATIVE

Social History:

_____

Cigs: [] No Yes [] → Pack yrs _____
ETOH [] No Yes [] → Amount? _____
Illicits [] No Yes [] → Type? _____
Allergies: [] NKDA _____
Medications:

_____
_____
_____
_____
_____
_____
_____
_____
_____
_____
_____

Physical Exam T _____ BP _____ HR _____ Wt _____(lbs) Ht _____(in) BMI _____

Eyes	[] nl conjunctiva & lids	**ENT** External	[] no scars, lesions, masses	**Neck** External	[]	no tracheal deviation	
Pupils	[] equal, round, & reactive	Otoscopic	[] nl canals, TM	Palpation	[]	no masses	
Fundus	[] nl discs and vessels	Hearing	[] nl hearing	Thyroid	[]	no enlargement	
Vision	[] acuity & gross fields intact	Oropharynx	[] nl teeth, tongue, pharynx	Abnormals:			
Abnormals:		Abnormals:					

GI Palpation [] no masses or tenderness	[] no hep/splenomegaly	**Resp** Effort	[] nl w/o retractions	**Skin**	[] no rashes, or lesions
Ausculation	[] nl bowel sounds	Percussion	[] no dullness	Chest	[] nl breast, no d/c
Percussion	[] no dullness	Palpation	[] no fremitus	Lymph nodes [] no axillary, inguinal, cervical or submandibular LAD	
Anus/rectum	[] no abnormality or masses	Ausculation	[] CTA w/o W, R, or R		
	[] heme negative stool	Abnormals:		GU	[] nl male/female exam
Abnormals:				Psych	[] nl cognition

CV Palpation [] PMI nondisplaced		**Neuro** Orientation [] AAO x 3		Abnormals:
Auscultation	[] no murmur, gallop, or rub	Cranial nerves	[] CN II-XII intact	
Carotids	[] nl intensity w/o bruit	Sensory	[] nl sensation	
JVD	[] no jugulovenous distention	Reflexes	[] 2+ & symmetrical	
Pulses	[] 2+/= femoral & pedal pulses	Abnormals:		
Edema	[] no pedal edema			
Abnormals				

Musculoskeletal Inspection ROM Strength Tone (✓ if normal) Abnormals: | **Other:**

	Inspection	ROM	Strength	Tone
Upper extremity	[]	[]	[]	[]
Lower extremity	[]	[]	[]	[]

Gait [] nl gait and FROM

Labs:

Assessment & Plan:

_____
_____
_____
_____
_____
_____
_____
_____
_____
_____
_____

Clinical Rotation_____   Date: _____

Chief Complaint:

_____

History of Present Illness:

_____
_____
_____
_____
_____

Review of Systems:

	Yes	No		Yes	No		Yes	No		Yes	No
General: fatigue	[]	[]	CV: chest pain	[]	[]	Bloody stool	[]	[]	Polydypsia	[]	[]
Weight loss	[]	[]	Edema	[]	[]	GU: dysuria	[]	[]	Polyphagia	[]	[]
Fever	[]	[]	PND	[]	[]	Frequency	[]	[]	Polyphagia	[]	[]
Chills	[]	[]	Orthopnea	[]	[]	Hematuria	[]	[]	Temp int	[]	[]
Night sweats	[]	[]	Palpitations	[]	[]	Discharge	[]	[]	Derm: rash	[]	[]
Eye: vision change	[]	[]	Claudication	[]	[]	Flank pain	[]	[]	Pruritis	[]	[]
Pain	[]	[]	Resp: cough	[]	[]	MS: arthralgia	[]	[]	Neuro: weakness	[]	[]
Redness	[]	[]	SOB	[]	[]	Arthritis	[]	[]	Seizures	[]	[]
ENT: headaches	[]	[]	Wheezing	[]	[]	Joint swelling	[]	[]	Parasthesias	[]	[]
Hoarseness	[]	[]	Hemoptysis	[]	[]	Myalgias	[]	[]	Tremors	[]	[]
Sore throat	[]	[]	GI: abd pain	[]	[]	Back pain	[]	[]	Syncope	[]	[]
Epistaxis	[]	[]	BM changes	[]	[]	Heme: bleeding	[]	[]	Psych: anxiety	[]	[]
Sinus Sx	[]	[]	N/V	[]	[]	Bruising	[]	[]	Depression	[]	[]
Hearing loss	[]	[]	Diarrhea	[]	[]	Lymph: swelling	[]	[]	Hallucinations	[]	[]
Tinnitus	[]	[]	Heartburn	[]	[]	Endo: polyuria	[]	[]	All/Imm: hayfever	[]	[]
									Runny nose	[]	[]

Other ROS: _____   [] All other ROS reviewed and were NEGATIVE

Past Medical History: **Social History:**

_____   _____
_____
_____   Cigs: [] No Yes [] → Pack yrs _____
_____   ETOH [] No Yes [] → Amount? _____
_____   Illicits [] No Yes [] → Type? _____
_____   **Allergies**: [] NKDA _____
                                         Medications:

Past Surgical History:

_____   _____
_____   _____
_____   _____
_____   _____

Family History: _____

_____   _____
_____   _____
_____   _____

Physical Exam T _____ BP _____ HR _____ Wt _____(lbs) Ht _____(in) BMI _____		
Eyes [] nl conjunctiva & lids	**ENT** External [] no scars, lesions, masses	**Neck** External [] no tracheal deviation
Pupils [] equal, round, & reactive	Otoscopic [] nl canals, TM	Palpation [] no masses
Fundus [] nl discs and vessels	Hearing [] nl hearing	Thyroid [] no enlargement
Vision [] acuity & gross fields intact	Oropharynx [] nl teeth, tongue, pharynx	Abnormals:
Abnormals:	Abnormals:	
GI Palpation [] no masses or tenderness [] no hep/splenomegaly	**Resp** Effort [] nl w/o retractions	**Skin** [] no rashes, or lesions
	Percussion [] no dullness	Chest [] nl breast, no d/c
Ausculation [] nl bowel sounds	Palpation [] no fremitus	Lymph nodes [] no axillary, inguinal, cervical or submandibular LAD
Percussion [] no dullness	Ausculation [] CTA w/o W, R, or R	
Anus/rectum [] no abnormality or masses [] heme negative stool	Abnormals:	GU [] nl male/female exam
Abnormals:		Psych [] nl cognition
CV Palpation [] PMI nondisplaced	**Neuro** Orientation [] AAO x 3	Abnormals:
Auscultation [] no murmur, gallop, or rub	Cranial nerves [] CN II-XII intact	
Carotids [] nl intensity w/o bruit	Sensory [] nl sensation	
JVD [] no jugulovenous distention	Reflexes [] 2+ & symmetrical	
Pulses [] 2+/= femoral & pedal pulses	Abnormals:	
Edema [] no pedal edema		
Abnormals		
Musculoskeletal Inspection ROM Strength Tone (✓ if normal) Abnormals:		**Other:**
Upper extremity [] [] [] [] Lower extremity [] [] [] []		
Gait [] nl gait and FROM		

Labs:

Assessment & Plan:
_____
_____
_____
_____
_____
_____
_____
_____
_____
_____

Clinical Rotation_____   Date: _____

Chief Complaint:
_____

History of Present Illness:
_____
_____
_____
_____
_____

Review of Systems:

	Yes	No		Yes	No		Yes	No		Yes	No
General: fatigue	[]	[]	CV: chest pain	[]	[]	Bloody stool	[]	[]	Polydypsia	[]	[]
Weight loss	[]	[]	Edema	[]	[]	GU: dysuria	[]	[]	Polyphagia	[]	[]
Fever	[]	[]	PND	[]	[]	Frequency	[]	[]	Polyphagia	[]	[]
Chills	[]	[]	Orthopnea	[]	[]	Hematuria	[]	[]	Temp int	[]	[]
Night sweats	[]	[]	Palpitations	[]	[]	Discharge	[]	[]	Derm: rash	[]	[]
Eye: vision change	[]	[]	Claudication	[]	[]	Flank pain	[]	[]	Neuro: weakness	[]	[]
Pain	[]	[]	Resp: cough	[]	[]	MS: arthralgia	[]	[]	Pruritis	[]	[]
Redness	[]	[]	SOB	[]	[]	Arthritis	[]	[]	Seizures	[]	[]
ENT: headaches	[]	[]	Wheezing	[]	[]	Joint swelling	[]	[]	Parasthesias	[]	[]
Hoarseness	[]	[]	Hemoptysis	[]	[]	Myalgias	[]	[]	Tremors	[]	[]
Sore throat	[]	[]	GI: abd pain	[]	[]	Back pain	[]	[]	Syncope	[]	[]
Epistaxis	[]	[]	BM changes	[]	[]	Heme: bleeding	[]	[]	Psych: anxiety	[]	[]
Sinus Sx	[]	[]	N/V	[]	[]	Bruising	[]	[]	Depression	[]	[]
Hearing loss	[]	[]	Diarrhea	[]	[]	Lymph: swelling	[]	[]	Hallucinations	[]	[]
Tinnitus	[]	[]	Heartburn	[]	[]	Endo: polyuria	[]	[]	All/Imm: hayfever	[]	[]
									Runny nose	[]	[]

Other ROS: _____

Past Medical History:
_____
_____
_____
_____
_____
_____

Past Surgical History:
_____
_____
_____
_____

Family History:
_____
_____
_____
_____

Social History:
_____

Cigs: [] No Yes [] → Pack yrs _____
ETOH [] No Yes [] → Amount? _____
Illicits [] No Yes [] → Type? _____
Allergies: [] NKDA _____
Medications:
_____
_____
_____
_____
_____
_____
_____
_____

[] All other ROS reviewed and were NEGATIVE

Physical Exam T _____ BP _____ HR _____ Wt _____ (lbs) Ht _____ (in) BMI _____

Eyes [] nl conjunctiva & lids	**ENT** External [] no scars, lesions, masses	**Neck** External [] no tracheal deviation
Pupils [] equal, round, & reactive	Otoscopic [] nl canals, TM	Palpation [] no masses
Fundus [] nl discs and vessels	Hearing [] nl hearing	Thyroid [] no enlargement
Vision [] acuity & gross fields intact	Oropharynx [] nl teeth, tongue, pharynx	Abnormals:
Abnormals:	Abnormals:	

GI Palpation [] no masses or tenderness [] no hep/splenomegaly	**Resp** Effort [] nl w/o retractions	**Skin** [] no rashes, or lesions
Ausculation [] nl bowel sounds	Percussion [] no dullness	Chest [] nl breast, no d/c
Percussion [] no dullness	Palpation [] no fremitus	Lymph nodes [] no axillary, inguinal, cervical or submandibular LAD
Anus/rectum [] no abnormality or masses [] heme negative stool	Ausculation [] CTA w/o W, R, or R	GU [] nl male/female exam
Abnormals:	Abnormals:	Psych [] nl cognition

CV Palpation [] PMI nondisplaced	**Neuro** Orientation [] AAO x 3	Abnormals:
Auscultation [] no murmur, gallop, or rub	Cranial nerves [] CN II-XII intact	
Carotids [] nl intensity w/o bruit	Sensory [] nl sensation	
JVD [] no jugulovenous distention	Reflexes [] 2+ & symmetrical	
Pulses [] 2+/= femoral & pedal pulses	Abnormals:	
Edema [] no pedal edema		
Abnormals		

Musculoskeletal Inspection ROM Strength Tone (✓ if normal) Abnormals: **Other:**

	Inspection	ROM	Strength	Tone
Upper extremity	[]	[]	[]	[]
Lower extremity	[]	[]	[]	[]

Gait [] nl gait and FROM

Labs:

Assessment & Plan:

_____
_____
_____
_____
_____
_____
_____
_____
_____
_____
_____

Clinical Rotation_____　　　　　　　　　**Date:** _____

Chief Complaint:
_____

History of Present Illness:
_____
_____
_____
_____
_____

Review of Systems:

	Yes	No		Yes	No		Yes	No		Yes	No
General: fatigue	[]	[]	CV: chest pain	[]	[]	Bloody stool	[]	[]	Polydypsia	[]	[]
Weight loss	[]	[]	Edema	[]	[]	GU: dysuria	[]	[]	Polyphagia	[]	[]
Fever	[]	[]	PND	[]	[]	Frequency	[]	[]	Polyphagia	[]	[]
Chills	[]	[]	Orthopnea	[]	[]	Hematuria	[]	[]	Temp int	[]	[]
Night sweats	[]	[]	Palpitations	[]	[]	Discharge	[]	[]	Derm: rash	[]	[]
Eye: vision change	[]	[]	Claudication	[]	[]	Flank pain	[]	[]	Pruritis	[]	[]
Pain	[]	[]	Resp: cough	[]	[]	MS: arthralgia	[]	[]	Neuro: weakness	[]	[]
Redness	[]	[]	SOB	[]	[]	Arthritis	[]	[]	Seizures	[]	[]
ENT: headaches	[]	[]	Wheezing	[]	[]	Joint swelling	[]	[]	Parasthesias	[]	[]
Hoarseness	[]	[]	Hemoptysis	[]	[]	Myalgias	[]	[]	Tremors	[]	[]
Sore throat	[]	[]	GI: abd pain	[]	[]	Back pain	[]	[]	Syncope	[]	[]
Epistaxis	[]	[]	BM changes	[]	[]	Heme: bleeding	[]	[]	Psych: anxiety	[]	[]
Sinus Sx	[]	[]	N/V	[]	[]	Bruising	[]	[]	Depression	[]	[]
Hearing loss	[]	[]	Diarrhea	[]	[]	Lymph: swelling	[]	[]	Hallucinations	[]	[]
Tinnitus	[]	[]	Heartburn	[]	[]	Endo: polyuria	[]	[]	All/Imm: hayfever	[]	[]
									Runny nose	[]	[]

Other ROS: _____

Past Medical History:
_____
_____
_____
_____
_____
_____
_____

Past Surgical History:
_____
_____
_____
_____

Family History:
_____
_____
_____

[] All other ROS reviewed and were NEGATIVE

Social History:
_____
_____

Cigs: [] No Yes [] → Pack yrs _____
ETOH [] No Yes [] → Amount? _____
Illicits [] No Yes [] → Type? _____
Allergies: [] NKDA _____
Medications:
_____
_____
_____
_____
_____
_____
_____
_____
_____

Physical Exam   T _____   BP _____   HR _____   Wt _____(lbs)   Ht _____(in)   BMI _____

Eyes			

Eyes	[] nl conjunctiva & lids	**ENT** External [] no scars, lesions, masses	**Neck** External [] no tracheal deviation
Pupils	[] equal, round, & reactive	Otoscopic [] nl canals, TM	Palpation [] no masses
Fundus	[] nl discs and vessels	Hearing [] nl hearing	Thyroid [] no enlargement
Vision	[] acuity & gross fields intact	Oropharynx [] nl teeth, tongue, pharynx	Abnormals:
Abnormals:		Abnormals:	
GI Palpation [] no masses or tenderness [] no hep/splenomegaly		**Resp** Effort [] nl w/o retractions	**Skin** [] no rashes, or lesions
Ausculation [] nl bowel sounds		Percussion [] no dullness	Chest [] nl breast, no d/c
Percussion [] no dullness		Palpation [] no fremitus	Lymph nodes [] no axillary, inguinal, cervical or submandibular LAD
Anus/rectum [] no abnormality or masses [] heme negative stool		Ausculation [] CTA w/o W, R, or R	GU [] nl male/female exam
Abnormals:		Abnormals:	Psych [] nl cognition
CV Palpation [] PMI nondisplaced		**Neuro** Orientation [] AAO x 3	Abnormals:
Auscultation [] no murmur, gallop, or rub		Cranial nerves [] CN II-XII intact	
Carotids [] nl intensity w/o bruit		Sensory [] nl sensation	
JVD [] no jugulovenous distention		Reflexes [] 2+ & symmetrical	
Pulses [] 2+/= femoral & pedal pulses		Abnormals:	
Edema [] no pedal edema			
Abnormals			

Musculoskeletal   Inspection   ROM   Strength   Tone   (✓ if normal)   Abnormals: **Other:**

Upper extremity   []   []   []   []
Lower extremity   []   []   []   []

Gait   []   nl gait and FROM

Labs:

>——< ——+——<

Assessment & Plan:

_____
_____
_____
_____
_____
_____
_____
_____
_____
_____
_____

Clinical Rotation_____   Date: _____

Chief Complaint:
_____

History of Present Illness:
_____
_____
_____
_____
_____

Review of Systems:

	Yes	No		Yes	No		Yes	No		Yes	No
General: fatigue	[]	[]	CV: chest pain	[]	[]	Bloody stool	[]	[]	Polydypsia	[]	[]
Weight loss	[]	[]	Edema	[]	[]	GU: dysuria	[]	[]	Polyphagia	[]	[]
Fever	[]	[]	PND	[]	[]	Frequency	[]	[]	Polyphagia	[]	[]
Chills	[]	[]	Orthopnea	[]	[]	Hematuria	[]	[]	Temp int	[]	[]
Night sweats	[]	[]	Palpitations	[]	[]	Discharge	[]	[]	Derm: rash	[]	[]
Eye: vision change	[]	[]	Claudication	[]	[]	Flank pain	[]	[]	Pruritis	[]	[]
Pain	[]	[]	Resp: cough	[]	[]	MS: arthralgia	[]	[]	Neuro: weakness	[]	[]
Redness	[]	[]	SOB	[]	[]	Arthritis	[]	[]	Seizures	[]	[]
ENT: headaches	[]	[]	Wheezing	[]	[]	Joint swelling	[]	[]	Parasthesias	[]	[]
Hoarseness	[]	[]	Hemoptysis	[]	[]	Myalgias	[]	[]	Tremors	[]	[]
Sore throat	[]	[]	GI: abd pain	[]	[]	Back pain	[]	[]	Syncope	[]	[]
Epistaxis	[]	[]	BM changes	[]	[]	Heme: bleeding	[]	[]	Psych: anxiety	[]	[]
Sinus Sx	[]	[]	N/V	[]	[]	Bruising	[]	[]	Depression	[]	[]
Hearing loss	[]	[]	Diarrhea	[]	[]	Lymph: swelling	[]	[]	Hallucinations	[]	[]
Tinnitus	[]	[]	Heartburn	[]	[]	Endo: polyuria	[]	[]	All/Imm: hayfever	[]	[]
									Runny nose	[]	[]

Other ROS: _____

Past Medical History:
_____
_____
_____
_____
_____
_____
_____

Past Surgical History:
_____
_____
_____
_____

Family History:
_____
_____
_____

[] All other ROS reviewed and were NEGATIVE

Social History:
_____
_____

Cigs: [] No Yes [] → Pack yrs _____
ETOH [] No Yes [] → Amount? _____
Illicits [] No Yes [] → Type? _____
Allergies: [] NKDA _____
Medications:
_____
_____
_____
_____
_____
_____
_____
_____
_____

Physical Exam T _____ BP _____ HR _____ Wt _____(lbs) Ht _____(in) BMI _____		
Eyes [] nl conjunctiva & lids	**ENT** External [] no scars, lesions, masses	**Neck** External [] no tracheal deviation
Pupils [] equal, round, & reactive	Otoscopic [] nl canals, TM	Palpation [] no masses
Fundus [] nl discs and vessels	Hearing [] nl hearing	Thyroid [] no enlargement
Vision [] acuity & gross fields intact	Oropharynx [] nl teeth, tongue, pharynx	Abnormals:
Abnormals:	Abnormals:	
GI Palpation [] no masses or tenderness [] no hep/splenomegaly	**Resp** Effort [] nl w/o retractions	**Skin** [] no rashes, or lesions
Ausculation [] nl bowel sounds	Percussion [] no dullness	Chest [] nl breast, no d/c
Percussion [] no dullness	Palpation [] no fremitus	Lymph nodes [] no axillary, inguinal, cervical or submandibular LAD
Anus/rectum [] no abnormality or masses [] heme negative stool	Ausculation [] CTA w/o W, R, or R	GU [] nl male/female exam
Abnormals:	Abnormals:	Psych [] nl cognition
CV Palpation [] PMI nondisplaced	**Neuro** Orientation [] AAO x 3	Abnormals:
Auscultation [] no murmur, gallop, or rub	Cranial nerves [] CN II-XII intact	
Carotids [] nl intensity w/o bruit	Sensory [] nl sensation	
JVD [] no jugulovenous distention	Reflexes [] 2+ & symmetrical	
Pulses [] 2+/= femoral & pedal pulses	Abnormals:	
Edema [] no pedal edema		
Abnormals		

Musculoskeletal Inspection ROM Strength Tone (✓ if normal) Abnormals:	**Other:**
Upper extremity [] [] [] [] Lower extremity [] [] [] []	
Gait [] nl gait and FROM	

Labs:

Assessment & Plan:

_____
_____
_____
_____
_____
_____
_____
_____
_____
_____
_____

Clinical Rotation_____   Date: _____

Chief Complaint:
_____

History of Present Illness:
_____
_____
_____
_____
_____

Review of Systems:

	Yes	No		Yes	No		Yes	No		Yes	No
General: fatigue	[]	[]	CV: chest pain	[]	[]	Bloody stool	[]	[]	Polydypsia	[]	[]
Weight loss	[]	[]	Edema	[]	[]	GU: dysuria	[]	[]	Polyphagia	[]	[]
Fever	[]	[]	PND	[]	[]	Frequency	[]	[]	Polyphagia	[]	[]
Chills	[]	[]	Orthopnea	[]	[]	Hematuria	[]	[]	Temp int	[]	[]
Night sweats	[]	[]	Palpitations	[]	[]	Discharge	[]	[]	Derm: rash	[]	[]
Eye: vision change	[]	[]	Claudication	[]	[]	Flank pain	[]	[]	Pruritis	[]	[]
Pain	[]	[]	Resp: cough	[]	[]	MS: arthralgia	[]	[]	Neuro: weakness	[]	[]
Redness	[]	[]	SOB	[]	[]	Arthritis	[]	[]	Seizures	[]	[]
ENT: headaches	[]	[]	Wheezing	[]	[]	Joint swelling	[]	[]	Parasthesias	[]	[]
Hoarseness	[]	[]	Hemoptysis	[]	[]	Myalgias	[]	[]	Tremors	[]	[]
Sore throat	[]	[]	GI: abd pain	[]	[]	Back pain	[]	[]	Syncope	[]	[]
Epistaxis	[]	[]	BM changes	[]	[]	Heme: bleeding	[]	[]	Psych: anxiety	[]	[]
Sinus Sx	[]	[]	N/V	[]	[]	Bruising	[]	[]	Depression	[]	[]
Hearing loss	[]	[]	Diarrhea	[]	[]	Lymph: swelling	[]	[]	Hallucinations	[]	[]
Tinnitus	[]	[]	Heartburn	[]	[]	Endo: polyuria	[]	[]	All/Imm: hayfever	[]	[]
									Runny nose	[]	[]

Other ROS: _____

Past Medical History:
_____
_____
_____
_____
_____
_____
_____

Past Surgical History:
_____
_____
_____
_____

Family History:
_____
_____

[] All other ROS reviewed and were NEGATIVE

Social History:
_____

Cigs: [] No Yes [] → Pack yrs _____
ETOH [] No Yes [] → Amount? _____
Illicits [] No Yes [] → Type? _____
Allergies: [] NKDA _____
Medications:
_____
_____
_____
_____
_____
_____
_____
_____
_____
_____

| Physical Exam   T _____   BP _____   HR _____   Wt _____(lbs)   Ht _____(in)   BMI _____ |

Eyes [] nl conjunctiva & lids	**ENT** External [] no scars, lesions, masses	**Neck** External [] no tracheal deviation
Pupils [] equal, round, & reactive	Otoscopic [] nl canals, TM	Palpation [] no masses
Fundus [] nl discs and vessels	Hearing [] nl hearing	Thyroid [] no enlargement
Vision [] acuity & gross fields intact	Oropharynx [] nl teeth, tongue, pharynx	Abnormals:
Abnormals:	Abnormals:	
GI Palpation [] no masses or tenderness [] no hep/splenomegaly	**Resp** Effort [] nl w/o retractions	**Skin** [] no rashes, or lesions
Ausculation [] nl bowel sounds	Percussion [] no dullness	Chest [] nl breast, no d/c
Percussion [] no dullness	Palpation [] no fremitus	Lymph nodes [] no axillary, inguinal, cervical or submandibular LAD
Anus/rectum [] no abnormality or masses [] heme negative stool	Ausculation [] CTA w/o W, R, or R	GU [] nl male/female exam
Abnormals:	Abnormals:	Psych [] nl cognition
CV Palpation [] PMI nondisplaced	**Neuro** Orientation [] AAO x 3	Abnormals:
Auscultation [] no murmur, gallop, or rub	Cranial nerves [] CN II-XII intact	
Carotids [] nl intensity w/o bruit	Sensory [] nl sensation	
JVD [] no jugulovenous distention	Reflexes [] 2+ & symmetrical	
Pulses [] 2+/= femoral & pedal pulses	Abnormals:	
Edema [] no pedal edema		
Abnormals		

Musculoskeletal Inspection ROM Strength Tone (✓ if normal) Abnormals:	**Other:**
Upper extremity [] [] [] [] Lower extremity [] [] [] [] Gait [] nl gait and FROM	

Labs:

Assessment & Plan:

_____

_____

_____

_____

_____

_____

_____

_____

_____

_____

_____

Clinical Rotation_____   Date: _____

Chief Complaint:
_____

History of Present Illness:
_____
_____
_____
_____
_____

Review of Systems:

	Yes	No		Yes	No		Yes	No		Yes	No
General: fatigue	[]	[]	CV: chest pain	[]	[]	Bloody stool	[]	[]	Polydypsia	[]	[]
Weight loss	[]	[]	Edema	[]	[]	GU: dysuria	[]	[]	Polyphagia	[]	[]
Fever	[]	[]	PND	[]	[]	Frequency	[]	[]	Polyphagia	[]	[]
Chills	[]	[]	Orthopnea	[]	[]	Hematuria	[]	[]	Temp int	[]	[]
Night sweats	[]	[]	Palpitations	[]	[]	Discharge	[]	[]	Derm: rash	[]	[]
Eye: vision change	[]	[]	Claudication	[]	[]	Flank pain	[]	[]	Pruritis	[]	[]
Pain	[]	[]	Resp: cough	[]	[]	MS: arthralgia	[]	[]	Neuro: weakness	[]	[]
Redness	[]	[]	SOB	[]	[]	Arthritis	[]	[]	Seizures	[]	[]
ENT: headaches	[]	[]	Wheezing	[]	[]	Joint swelling	[]	[]	Parasthesias	[]	[]
Hoarseness	[]	[]	Hemoptysis	[]	[]	Myalgias	[]	[]	Tremors	[]	[]
Sore throat	[]	[]	GI: abd pain	[]	[]	Back pain	[]	[]	Syncope	[]	[]
Epistaxis	[]	[]	BM changes	[]	[]	Heme: bleeding	[]	[]	Psych: anxiety	[]	[]
Sinus Sx	[]	[]	N/V	[]	[]	Bruising	[]	[]	Depression	[]	[]
Hearing loss	[]	[]	Diarrhea	[]	[]	Lymph: swelling	[]	[]	Hallucinations	[]	[]
Tinnitus	[]	[]	Heartburn	[]	[]	Endo: polyuria	[]	[]	All/Imm: hayfever	[]	[]
									Runny nose	[]	[]

Other ROS: _____

Past Medical History:
_____
_____
_____
_____
_____
_____
_____

Past Surgical History:
_____
_____
_____
_____

Family History:
_____
_____
_____

[] All other ROS reviewed and were NEGATIVE

Social History:
_____

Cigs: [] No Yes [] → Pack yrs _____
ETOH [] No Yes [] → Amount? _____
Illicits [] No Yes [] → Type? _____
Allergies: [] NKDA _____
Medications:
_____
_____
_____
_____
_____
_____
_____
_____
_____
_____
_____

Physical Exam	T _____	BP _____	HR _____	Wt _____(lbs)	Ht _____(in)	BMI _____

Eyes	[] nl conjunctiva & lids	ENT External	[] no scars, lesions, masses	Neck External	[] no tracheal deviation
Pupils	[] equal, round, & reactive	Otoscopic	[] nl canals, TM	Palpation	[] no masses
Fundus	[] nl discs and vessels	Hearing	[] nl hearing	Thyroid	[] no enlargement
Vision	[] acuity & gross fields intact	Oropharynx	[] nl teeth, tongue, pharynx	Abnormals:	
Abnormals:		Abnormals:			

GI Palpation	[] no masses or tenderness [] no hep/splenomegaly	Resp Effort	[] nl w/o retractions	Skin	[] no rashes, or lesions
		Percussion	[] no dullness	Chest	[] nl breast, no d/c
Ausculation	[] nl bowel sounds	Palpation	[] no fremitus	Lymph nodes	[] no axillary, inguinal, cervical or submandibular LAD
Percussion	[] no dullness	Ausculation	[] CTA w/o W, R, or R		
Anus/rectum	[] no abnormality or masses [] heme negative stool	Abnormals:		GU	[] nl male/female exam
Abnormals:				Psych	[] nl cognition

CV Palpation	[] PMI nondisplaced	Neuro Orientation	[] AAO x 3	Abnormals:	
Auscultation	[] no murmur, gallop, or rub	Cranial nerves	[] CN II-XII intact		
Carotids	[] nl intensity w/o bruit	Sensory	[] nl sensation		
JVD	[] no jugulovenous distention	Reflexes	[] 2+ & symmetrical		
Pulses	[] 2+/= femoral & pedal pulses	Abnormals:			
Edema	[] no pedal edema				
Abnormals					

Musculoskeletal	Inspection	ROM	Strength	Tone (✓ if normal)	Abnormals:	Other:
Upper extremity	[]	[]	[]	[]		
Lower extremity	[]	[]	[]	[]		
Gait	[] nl gait and FROM					

Labs:

Assessment & Plan:

_____
_____
_____
_____
_____
_____
_____
_____
_____
_____

Clinical Rotation_____   Date: _____

Chief Complaint:

_____

History of Present Illness:

_____
_____
_____
_____
_____

Review of Systems:

	Yes No		Yes No		Yes No		Yes No
General: fatigue	[] []	CV: chest pain	[] []	Bloody stool	[] []	Polydypsia	[] []
Weight loss	[] []	Edema	[] []	GU: dysuria	[] []	Polyphagia	[] []
Fever	[] []	PND	[] []	Frequency	[] []	Polyphagia	[] []
Chills	[] []	Orthopnea	[] []	Hematuria	[] []	Temp int	[] []
Night sweats	[] []	Palpitations	[] []	Discharge	[] []	Derm: rash	[] []
Eye: vision change	[] []	Claudication	[] []	Flank pain	[] []	Pruritis	[] []
Pain	[] []	Resp: cough	[] []	MS: arthralgia	[] []	Neuro: weakness	[] []
Redness	[] []	SOB	[] []	Arthritis	[] []	Seizures	[] []
ENT: headaches	[] []	Wheezing	[] []	Joint swelling	[] []	Parasthesias	[] []
Hoarseness	[] []	Hemoptysis	[] []	Myalgias	[] []	Tremors	[] []
Sore throat	[] []	GI: abd pain	[] []	Back pain	[] []	Syncope	[] []
Epistaxis	[] []	BM changes	[] []	Heme: bleeding	[] []	Psych: anxiety	[] []
Sinus Sx	[] []	N/V	[] []	Bruising	[] []	Depression	[] []
Hearing loss	[] []	Diarrhea	[] []	Lymph: swelling	[] []	Hallucinations	[] []
Tinnitus	[] []	Heartburn	[] []	Endo: polyuria	[] []	All/Imm: hayfever	[] []
						Runny nose	[] []

Other ROS: _____

Past Medical History:

_____
_____
_____
_____
_____
_____

Past Surgical History:

_____
_____
_____
_____

Family History:

_____
_____
_____

[] All other ROS reviewed and were NEGATIVE

Social History:

_____

Cigs: [] No Yes [] → Pack yrs _____
ETOH [] No Yes [] → Amount? _____
Illicits [] No Yes [] → Type? _____
Allergies: [] NKDA _____
Medications:

_____
_____
_____
_____
_____
_____
_____
_____
_____

Physical Exam T _____ BP _____ HR _____ Wt _____(lbs) Ht _____(in) BMI _____

Eyes		**ENT** External	[] no scars, lesions, masses	**Neck** External	[] no tracheal deviation
Eyes	[] nl conjunctiva & lids				
Pupils	[] equal, round, & reactive	Otoscopic	[] nl canals, TM	Palpation	[] no masses
Fundus	[] nl discs and vessels	Hearing	[] nl hearing	Thyroid	[] no enlargement
Vision	[] acuity & gross fields intact	Oropharynx	[] nl teeth, tongue, pharynx	Abnormals:	
Abnormals:		Abnormals:			

GI Palpation	[] no masses or tenderness	**Resp** Effort	[] nl w/o retractions	**Skin**	[] no rashes, or lesions
	[] no hep/splenomegaly	Percussion	[] no dullness	Chest	[] nl breast, no d/c
Ausculation	[] nl bowel sounds	Palpation	[] no fremitus	Lymph nodes	[] no axillary, inguinal, cervical or submandibular LAD
Percussion	[] no dullness	Ausculation	[] CTA w/o W, R, or R		
Anus/rectum	[] no abnormality or masses	Abnormals:		GU	[] nl male/female exam
	[] heme negative stool			Psych	[] nl cognition
Abnormals:				Abnormals:	

CV Palpation	[] PMI nondisplaced	**Neuro** Orientation	[] AAO x 3		
Auscultation	[] no murmur, gallop, or rub	Cranial nerves	[] CN II-XII intact		
Carotids	[] nl intensity w/o bruit	Sensory	[] nl sensation		
JVD	[] no jugulovenous distention	Reflexes	[] 2+ & symmetrical		
Pulses	[] 2+/= femoral & pedal pulses	Abnormals:			
Edema	[] no pedal edema				
Abnormals					

Musculoskeletal	Inspection	ROM	Strength	Tone (✓ if normal)	Abnormals:	**Other:**
Upper extremity	[]	[]	[]	[]		
Lower extremity	[]	[]	[]	[]		
Gait	[] nl gait and FROM					

Labs:

Assessment & Plan:

_____
_____
_____
_____
_____
_____
_____
_____
_____
_____
_____
_____

Clinical Rotation_____   Date: _____

Chief Complaint:
_____

History of Present Illness:
_____
_____
_____
_____
_____

Review of Systems:

	Yes	No		Yes	No		Yes	No		Yes	No
General: fatigue	[]	[]	CV: chest pain	[]	[]	Bloody stool	[]	[]	Polydypsia	[]	[]
Weight loss	[]	[]	Edema	[]	[]	GU: dysuria	[]	[]	Polyphagia	[]	[]
Fever	[]	[]	PND	[]	[]	Frequency	[]	[]	Polyphagia	[]	[]
Chills	[]	[]	Orthopnea	[]	[]	Hematuria	[]	[]	Temp int	[]	[]
Night sweats	[]	[]	Palpitations	[]	[]	Discharge	[]	[]	Derm: rash	[]	[]
Eye: vision change	[]	[]	Claudication	[]	[]	Flank pain	[]	[]	Pruritis	[]	[]
Pain	[]	[]	Resp: cough	[]	[]	MS: arthralgia	[]	[]	Neuro: weakness	[]	[]
Redness	[]	[]	SOB	[]	[]	Arthritis	[]	[]	Seizures	[]	[]
ENT: headaches	[]	[]	Wheezing	[]	[]	Joint swelling	[]	[]	Parasthesias	[]	[]
Hoarseness	[]	[]	Hemoptysis	[]	[]	Myalgias	[]	[]	Tremors	[]	[]
Sore throat	[]	[]	GI: abd pain	[]	[]	Back pain	[]	[]	Syncope	[]	[]
Epistaxis	[]	[]	BM changes	[]	[]	Heme: bleeding	[]	[]	Psych: anxiety	[]	[]
Sinus Sx	[]	[]	N/V	[]	[]	Bruising	[]	[]	Depression	[]	[]
Hearing loss	[]	[]	Diarrhea	[]	[]	Lymph: swelling	[]	[]	Hallucinations	[]	[]
Tinnitus	[]	[]	Heartburn	[]	[]	Endo: polyuria	[]	[]	All/Imm: hayfever	[]	[]
									Runny nose	[]	[]

Other ROS: _____

Past Medical History:
_____
_____
_____
_____
_____
_____

Past Surgical History:
_____
_____
_____
_____

Family History:
_____
_____

[] All other ROS reviewed and were NEGATIVE

Social History:
_____

Cigs: [] No Yes [] → Pack yrs _____
ETOH [] No Yes [] → Amount? _____
Illicits [] No Yes [] → Type? _____
Allergies: [] NKDA _____
Medications:
_____
_____
_____
_____
_____
_____
_____
_____
_____
_____

| Physical Exam | T _____ | BP _____ | HR _____ | Wt _____(lbs) | Ht _____(in) | BMI _____ |

Eyes	[] nl conjunctiva & lids	ENT External	[] no scars, lesions, masses	Neck External	[] no tracheal deviation
Pupils	[] equal, round, & reactive	Otoscopic	[] nl canals, TM	Palpation	[] no masses
Fundus	[] nl discs and vessels	Hearing	[] nl hearing	Thyroid	[] no enlargement
Vision	[] acuity & gross fields intact	Oropharynx	[] nl teeth, tongue, pharynx	Abnormals:	
Abnormals:		Abnormals:			

GI Palpation	[] no masses or tenderness [] no hep/splenomegaly	**Resp** Effort	[] nl w/o retractions	**Skin**	[] no rashes, or lesions
Ausculation	[] nl bowel sounds	Percussion	[] no dullness	Chest	[] nl breast, no d/c
Percussion	[] no dullness	Palpation	[] no fremitus	Lymph nodes	[] no axillary, inguinal, cervical or submandibular LAD
Anus/rectum	[] no abnormality or masses [] heme negative stool	Ausculation	[] CTA w/o W, R, or R	GU	[] nl male/female exam
Abnormals:		Abnormals:		Psych	[] nl cognition

CV Palpation	[] PMI nondisplaced	**Neuro** Orientation	[] AAO x 3	Abnormals:	
Auscultation	[] no murmur, gallop, or rub	Cranial nerves	[] CN II-XII intact		
Carotids	[] nl intensity w/o bruit	Sensory	[] nl sensation		
JVD	[] no jugulovenous distention	Reflexes	[] 2+ & symmetrical		
Pulses	[] 2+/= femoral & pedal pulses	Abnormals:			
Edema	[] no pedal edema				
Abnormals					

Musculoskeletal	Inspection	ROM	Strength	Tone (✓ if normal)	Abnormals:	**Other:**
Upper extremity	[]	[]	[]	[]		
Lower extremity	[]	[]	[]	[]		
Gait	[] nl gait and FROM					

Labs:

Assessment & Plan:

_____
_____
_____
_____
_____
_____
_____
_____
_____
_____

Clinical Rotation_____   Date: _____

Chief Complaint:
_____

History of Present Illness:
_____
_____
_____
_____
_____

Review of Systems:

	Yes	No		Yes	No		Yes	No		Yes	No
General: fatigue	[]	[]	CV: chest pain	[]	[]	Bloody stool	[]	[]	Polydypsia	[]	[]
Weight loss	[]	[]	Edema	[]	[]	GU: dysuria	[]	[]	Polyphagia	[]	[]
Fever	[]	[]	PND	[]	[]	Frequency	[]	[]	Polyphagia	[]	[]
Chills	[]	[]	Orthopnea	[]	[]	Hematuria	[]	[]	Temp int	[]	[]
Night sweats	[]	[]	Palpitations	[]	[]	Discharge	[]	[]	Derm: rash	[]	[]
Eye: vision change	[]	[]	Claudication	[]	[]	Flank pain	[]	[]	Pruritis	[]	[]
Pain	[]	[]	Resp: cough	[]	[]	MS: arthralgia	[]	[]	Neuro: weakness	[]	[]
Redness	[]	[]	SOB	[]	[]	Arthritis	[]	[]	Seizures	[]	[]
ENT: headaches	[]	[]	Wheezing	[]	[]	Joint swelling	[]	[]	Parasthesias	[]	[]
Hoarseness	[]	[]	Hemoptysis	[]	[]	Myalgias	[]	[]	Tremors	[]	[]
Sore throat	[]	[]	GI: abd pain	[]	[]	Back pain	[]	[]	Syncope	[]	[]
Epistaxis	[]	[]	BM changes	[]	[]	Heme: bleeding	[]	[]	Psych: anxiety	[]	[]
Sinus Sx	[]	[]	N/V	[]	[]	Bruising	[]	[]	Depression	[]	[]
Hearing loss	[]	[]	Diarrhea	[]	[]	Lymph: swelling	[]	[]	Hallucinations	[]	[]
Tinnitus	[]	[]	Heartburn	[]	[]	Endo: polyuria	[]	[]	All/Imm: hayfever	[]	[]
									Runny nose	[]	[]

Other ROS: _____

Past Medical History:
_____
_____
_____
_____
_____
_____

Past Surgical History:
_____
_____
_____
_____

Family History:
_____
_____

[] All other ROS reviewed and were NEGATIVE

Social History:
_____

Cigs: [] No Yes [] → Pack yrs _____
ETOH [] No Yes [] → Amount? _____
Illicits [] No Yes [] → Type? _____
Allergies: [] NKDA _____
Medications:
_____
_____
_____
_____
_____
_____
_____
_____
_____
_____
_____
_____

Physical Exam T _____ BP _____ HR _____ Wt _____(lbs) Ht _____(in) BMI _____

Eyes	[] nl conjunctiva & lids	**ENT** External	[] no scars, lesions, masses	**Neck** External	[] no tracheal deviation
Pupils	[] equal, round, & reactive	Otoscopic	[] nl canals, TM	Palpation	[] no masses
Fundus	[] nl discs and vessels	Hearing	[] nl hearing	Thyroid	[] no enlargement
Vision	[] acuity & gross fields intact	Oropharynx	[] nl teeth, tongue, pharynx	Abnormals:	
Abnormals:		Abnormals:			

GI Palpation []	no masses or tenderness	**Resp** Effort	[] nl w/o retractions	**Skin**	[] no rashes, or lesions
[]	no hep/splenomegaly	Percussion	[] no dullness	Chest	[] nl breast, no d/c
Ausculation []	nl bowel sounds	Palpation	[] no fremitus	Lymph nodes	[] no axillary, inguinal, cervical or submandibular LAD
Percussion []	no dullness	Ausculation	[] CTA w/o W, R, or R		
Anus/rectum []	no abnormality or masses	Abnormals:		GU	[] nl male/female exam
[]	heme negative stool				
Abnormals:				Psych	[] nl cognition

CV Palpation []	PMI nondisplaced	**Neuro** Orientation [] AAO x 3	Abnormals:
Auscultation []	no murmur, gallop, or rub	Cranial nerves [] CN II-XII intact	
Carotids []	nl intensity w/o bruit	Sensory [] nl sensation	
JVD []	no jugulovenous distention	Reflexes [] 2+ & symmetrical	
Pulses []	2+/= femoral & pedal pulses	Abnormals:	
Edema []	no pedal edema		
Abnormals			

Musculoskeletal Inspection ROM Strength Tone (✓ if normal) Abnormals:	**Other:**
Upper extremity [] [] [] []	
Lower extremity [] [] [] []	
Gait [] nl gait and FROM	

Labs:

Assessment & Plan:

_____
_____
_____
_____
_____
_____
_____
_____
_____
_____
_____

Clinical Rotation_____   Date: _____

Chief Complaint:
_____

History of Present Illness:
_____
_____
_____
_____
_____

Review of Systems:

	Yes No		Yes No		Yes No		Yes No
General: fatigue	[] []	CV: chest pain	[] []	Bloody stool	[] []	Polydypsia	[] []
Weight loss	[] []	Edema	[] []	GU: dysuria	[] []	Polyphagia	[] []
Fever	[] []	PND	[] []	Frequency	[] []	Polyphagia	[] []
Chills	[] []	Orthopnea	[] []	Hematuria	[] []	Temp int	[] []
Night sweats	[] []	Palpitations	[] []	Discharge	[] []	Derm: rash	[] []
Eye: vision change	[] []	Claudication	[] []	Flank pain	[] []	Pruritis	[] []
Pain	[] []	Resp: cough	[] []	MS: arthralgia	[] []	Neuro: weakness	[] []
Redness	[] []	SOB	[] []	Arthritis	[] []	Seizures	[] []
ENT: headaches	[] []	Wheezing	[] []	Joint swelling	[] []	Parasthesias	[] []
Hoarseness	[] []	Hemoptysis	[] []	Myalgias	[] []	Tremors	[] []
Sore throat	[] []	GI: abd pain	[] []	Back pain	[] []	Syncope	[] []
Epistaxis	[] []	BM changes	[] []	Heme: bleeding	[] []	Psych: anxiety	[] []
Sinus Sx	[] []	N/V	[] []	Bruising	[] []	Depression	[] []
Hearing loss	[] []	Diarrhea	[] []	Lymph: swelling	[] []	Hallucinations	[] []
Tinnitus	[] []	Heartburn	[] []	Endo: polyuria	[] []	All/Imm: hayfever	[] []
						Runny nose	[] []

Other ROS: _____

Past Medical History:
_____
_____
_____
_____
_____
_____

Past Surgical History:
_____
_____
_____
_____

Family History:
_____
_____

[ ] All other ROS reviewed and were NEGATIVE

Social History:
_____

Cigs: [] No Yes [] → Pack yrs _____
ETOH [] No Yes [] → Amount? _____
Illicits [] No Yes [] → Type? _____
Allergies: [] NKDA _____
Medications:
_____
_____
_____
_____
_____
_____
_____
_____
_____
_____

Physical Exam T _____ BP _____ HR _____ Wt _____(lbs) Ht _____(in) BMI _____		
Eyes [] nl conjunctiva & lids	**ENT** External [] no scars, lesions, masses	**Neck** External [] no tracheal deviation
Pupils [] equal, round, & reactive	Otoscopic [] nl canals, TM	Palpation [] no masses
Fundus [] nl discs and vessels	Hearing [] nl hearing	Thyroid [] no enlargement
Vision [] acuity & gross fields intact	Oropharynx [] nl teeth, tongue, pharynx	Abnormals:
Abnormals:	Abnormals:	
GI Palpation [] no masses or tenderness [] no hep/splenomegaly	**Resp** Effort [] nl w/o retractions	**Skin** [] no rashes, or lesions
	Percussion [] no dullness	Chest [] nl breast, no d/c
Ausculation [] nl bowel sounds	Palpation [] no fremitus	Lymph nodes [] no axillary, inguinal, cervical or submandibular LAD
Percussion [] no dullness	Ausculation [] CTA w/o W, R, or R	
Anus/rectum [] no abnormality or masses [] heme negative stool	Abnormals:	GU [] nl male/female exam
Abnormals:		Psych [] nl cognition
CV Palpation [] PMI nondisplaced	**Neuro** Orientation [] AAO x 3	Abnormals:
Auscultation [] no murmur, gallop, or rub	Cranial nerves [] CN II-XII intact	
Carotids [] nl intensity w/o bruit	Sensory [] nl sensation	
JVD [] no jugulovenous distention	Reflexes [] 2+ & symmetrical	
Pulses [] 2+/= femoral & pedal pulses	Abnormals:	
Edema [] no pedal edema		
Abnormals		

Musculoskeletal Inspection ROM Strength Tone (✓ if normal) Abnormals:	**Other:**
Upper extremity [] [] [] [] Lower extremity [] [] [] []	
Gait [] nl gait and FROM	

Labs:

Assessment & Plan:

_____
_____
_____
_____
_____
_____
_____
_____
_____
_____
_____

Clinical Rotation_____   Date: _____

Chief Complaint:
_____

History of Present Illness:
_____
_____
_____
_____
_____

Review of Systems:

	Yes No		Yes No		Yes No		Yes No
General: fatigue	[] []	CV: chest pain	[] []	Bloody stool	[] []	Polydypsia	[] []
Weight loss	[] []	Edema	[] []	GU: dysuria	[] []	Polyphagia	[] []
Fever	[] []	PND	[] []	Frequency	[] []	Polyphagia	[] []
Chills	[] []	Orthopnea	[] []	Hematuria	[] []	Temp int	[] []
Night sweats	[] []	Palpitations	[] []	Discharge	[] []	Derm: rash	[] []
Eye: vision change	[] []	Claudication	[] []	Flank pain	[] []	Pruritis	[] []
Pain	[] []	Resp: cough	[] []	MS: arthralgia	[] []	Neuro: weakness	[] []
Redness	[] []	SOB	[] []	Arthritis	[] []	Seizures	[] []
ENT: headaches	[] []	Wheezing	[] []	Joint swelling	[] []	Parasthesias	[] []
Hoarseness	[] []	Hemoptysis	[] []	Myalgias	[] []	Tremors	[] []
Sore throat	[] []	GI: abd pain	[] []	Back pain	[] []	Syncope	[] []
Epistaxis	[] []	BM changes	[] []	Heme: bleeding	[] []	Psych: anxiety	[] []
Sinus Sx	[] []	N/V	[] []	Bruising	[] []	Depression	[] []
Hearing loss	[] []	Diarrhea	[] []	Lymph: swelling	[] []	Hallucinations	[] []
Tinnitus	[] []	Heartburn	[] []	Endo: polyuria	[] []	All/Imm: hayfever	[] []
						Runny nose	[] []

Other ROS: _____

Past Medical History:
_____
_____
_____
_____
_____
_____

Social History:
_____

Cigs: [] No Yes [] → Pack yrs _____
ETOH [] No Yes [] → Amount? _____
Illicits [] No Yes [] → Type? _____
Allergies: [] NKDA _____
Medications:

Past Surgical History:
_____
_____
_____
_____

_____
_____
_____

Family History:
_____
_____

_____
_____
_____

[] All other ROS reviewed and were NEGATIVE

Physical Exam T _____ BP _____ HR _____ Wt _____ (lbs) Ht _____ (in) BMI _____		
Eyes [] nl conjunctiva & lids	**ENT** External [] no scars, lesions, masses	**Neck** External [] no tracheal deviation
Pupils [] equal, round, & reactive	Otoscopic [] nl canals, TM	Palpation [] no masses
Fundus [] nl discs and vessels	Hearing [] nl hearing	Thyroid [] no enlargement
Vision [] acuity & gross fields intact	Oropharynx [] nl teeth, tongue, pharynx	Abnormals:
Abnormals:	Abnormals:	
GI Palpation [] no masses or tenderness [] no hep/splenomegaly	**Resp** Effort [] nl w/o retractions	**Skin** [] no rashes, or lesions
Ausculation [] nl bowel sounds	Percussion [] no dullness	Chest [] nl breast, no d/c
Percussion [] no dullness	Palpation [] no fremitus	Lymph nodes [] no axillary, inguinal, cervical or submandibular LAD
Anus/rectum [] no abnormality or masses [] heme negative stool	Ausculation [] CTA w/o W, R, or R	GU [] nl male/female exam
Abnormals:	Abnormals:	Psych [] nl cognition
CV Palpation [] PMI nondisplaced	**Neuro** Orientation [] AAO x 3	Abnormals:
Auscultation [] no murmur, gallop, or rub	Cranial nerves [] CN II-XII intact	
Carotids [] nl intensity w/o bruit	Sensory [] nl sensation	
JVD [] no jugulovenous distention	Reflexes [] 2+ & symmetrical	
Pulses [] 2+/= femoral & pedal pulses	Abnormals:	
Edema [] no pedal edema		
Abnormals		
Musculoskeletal Inspection ROM Strength Tone (✓ if normal) Abnormals:		**Other:**
Upper extremity [] [] [] [] Lower extremity [] [] [] []		
Gait [] nl gait and FROM		

Labs:

Assessment & Plan:

Clinical Rotation_____   Date: _____

Chief Complaint:
_____

History of Present Illness:
_____
_____
_____
_____
_____

Review of Systems:

	Yes No		Yes No		Yes No		Yes No
General: fatigue	[] []	CV: chest pain	[] []	Bloody stool	[] []	Polydypsia	[] []
Weight loss	[] []	Edema	[] []	GU: dysuria	[] []	Polyphagia	[] []
Fever	[] []	PND	[] []	Frequency	[] []	Polyphagia	[] []
Chills	[] []	Orthopnea	[] []	Hematuria	[] []	Temp int	[] []
Night sweats	[] []	Palpitations	[] []	Discharge	[] []	Derm: rash	[] []
Eye: vision change	[] []	Claudication	[] []	Flank pain	[] []	Pruritis	[] []
Pain	[] []	Resp: cough	[] []	MS: arthralgia	[] []	Neuro: weakness	[] []
Redness	[] []	SOB	[] []	Arthritis	[] []	Seizures	[] []
ENT: headaches	[] []	Wheezing	[] []	Joint swelling	[] []	Parasthesias	[] []
Hoarseness	[] []	Hemoptysis	[] []	Myalgias	[] []	Tremors	[] []
Sore throat	[] []	GI: abd pain	[] []	Back pain	[] []	Syncope	[] []
Epistaxis	[] []	BM changes	[] []	Heme: bleeding	[] []	Psych: anxiety	[] []
Sinus Sx	[] []	N/V	[] []	Bruising	[] []	Depression	[] []
Hearing loss	[] []	Diarrhea	[] []	Lymph: swelling	[] []	Hallucinations	[] []
Tinnitus	[] []	Heartburn	[] []	Endo: polyuria	[] []	All/Imm: hayfever	[] []
						Runny nose	[] []

Other ROS: _____

Past Medical History:
_____
_____
_____
_____
_____
_____

Social History:
_____

Cigs: [] No Yes [] → Pack yrs _____
ETOH [] No Yes [] → Amount? _____
Illicits [] No Yes [] → Type? _____
Allergies: [] NKDA _____
Medications:
_____
_____

Past Surgical History:
_____
_____
_____
_____

_____
_____
_____
_____

Family History:
_____
_____
_____

_____
_____
_____

[] All other ROS reviewed and were NEGATIVE

Physical Exam T _____ BP _____ HR _____ Wt _____(lbs) Ht _____(in) BMI _____		
Eyes [] nl conjunctiva & lids	**ENT** External [] no scars, lesions, masses	**Neck** External [] no tracheal deviation
Pupils [] equal, round, & reactive	Otoscopic [] nl canals, TM	Palpation [] no masses
Fundus [] nl discs and vessels	Hearing [] nl hearing	Thyroid [] no enlargement
Vision [] acuity & gross fields intact	Oropharynx [] nl teeth, tongue, pharynx	Abnormals:
Abnormals:	Abnormals:	
GI Palpation [] no masses or tenderness [] no hep/splenomegaly	**Resp** Effort [] nl w/o retractions	**Skin** [] no rashes, or lesions
Ausculation [] nl bowel sounds	Percussion [] no dullness	Chest [] nl breast, no d/c
Percussion [] no dullness	Palpation [] no fremitus	Lymph nodes [] no axillary, inguinal, cervical or submandibular LAD
Anus/rectum [] no abnormality or masses [] heme negative stool	Ausculation [] CTA w/o W, R, or R Abnormals:	GU [] nl male/female exam
Abnormals:		Psych [] nl cognition
CV Palpation [] PMI nondisplaced	**Neuro** Orientation [] AAO x 3	Abnormals:
Auscultation [] no murmur, gallop, or rub	Cranial nerves [] CN II-XII intact	
Carotids [] nl intensity w/o bruit	Sensory [] nl sensation	
JVD [] no jugulovenous distention	Reflexes [] 2+ & symmetrical	
Pulses [] 2+/= femoral & pedal pulses	Abnormals:	
Edema [] no pedal edema		
Abnormals		

Musculoskeletal Inspection ROM Strength Tone (✓ if normal) Abnormals:	**Other:**
Upper extremity [] [] [] [] Lower extremity [] [] [] []	
Gait [] nl gait and FROM	

Labs:

Assessment & Plan:

_____
_____
_____
_____
_____
_____
_____
_____
_____
_____
_____

Clinical Rotation_____   Date: _____

Chief Complaint:
_____

History of Present Illness:
_____
_____
_____
_____
_____

Review of Systems:

	Yes	No		Yes	No		Yes	No		Yes	No
General: fatigue	[]	[]	CV: chest pain	[]	[]	Bloody stool	[]	[]	Polydypsia	[]	[]
Weight loss	[]	[]	Edema	[]	[]	GU: dysuria	[]	[]	Polyphagia	[]	[]
Fever	[]	[]	PND	[]	[]	Frequency	[]	[]	Polyphagia	[]	[]
Chills	[]	[]	Orthopnea	[]	[]	Hematuria	[]	[]	Temp int	[]	[]
Night sweats	[]	[]	Palpitations	[]	[]	Discharge	[]	[]	Derm: rash	[]	[]
Eye: vision change	[]	[]	Claudication	[]	[]	Flank pain	[]	[]	Pruritis	[]	[]
Pain	[]	[]	Resp: cough	[]	[]	MS: arthralgia	[]	[]	Neuro: weakness	[]	[]
Redness	[]	[]	SOB	[]	[]	Arthritis	[]	[]	Seizures	[]	[]
ENT: headaches	[]	[]	Wheezing	[]	[]	Joint swelling	[]	[]	Parasthesias	[]	[]
Hoarseness	[]	[]	Hemoptysis	[]	[]	Myalgias	[]	[]	Tremors	[]	[]
Sore throat	[]	[]	GI: abd pain	[]	[]	Back pain	[]	[]	Syncope	[]	[]
Epistaxis	[]	[]	BM changes	[]	[]	Heme: bleeding	[]	[]	Psych: anxiety	[]	[]
Sinus Sx	[]	[]	N/V	[]	[]	Bruising	[]	[]	Depression	[]	[]
Hearing loss	[]	[]	Diarrhea	[]	[]	Lymph: swelling	[]	[]	Hallucinations	[]	[]
Tinnitus	[]	[]	Heartburn	[]	[]	Endo: polyuria	[]	[]	All/Imm: hayfever	[]	[]
									Runny nose	[]	[]

Other ROS: _____

Past Medical History:
_____
_____
_____
_____
_____
_____
_____

Past Surgical History:
_____
_____
_____
_____

Family History:
_____
_____
_____

[] All other ROS reviewed and were NEGATIVE

Social History:
_____

Cigs: [] No Yes [] → Pack yrs _____
ETOH [] No Yes [] → Amount? _____
Illicits [] No Yes [] → Type? _____
Allergies: [] NKDA _____
Medications:
_____
_____
_____
_____
_____
_____
_____
_____
_____
_____
_____

Physical Exam T _____ BP _____ HR _____ Wt _____(lbs) Ht _____(in) BMI _____		
Eyes [] nl conjunctiva & lids	**ENT** External [] no scars, lesions, masses	**Neck** External [] no tracheal deviation
Pupils [] equal, round, & reactive	Otoscopic [] nl canals, TM	Palpation [] no masses
Fundus [] nl discs and vessels	Hearing [] nl hearing	Thyroid [] no enlargement
Vision [] acuity & gross fields intact	Oropharynx [] nl teeth, tongue, pharynx	Abnormals:
Abnormals:	Abnormals:	
GI Palpation [] no masses or tenderness [] no hep/splenomegaly	**Resp** Effort [] nl w/o retractions	**Skin** [] no rashes, or lesions
Ausculation [] nl bowel sounds	Percussion [] no dullness	Chest [] nl breast, no d/c
Percussion [] no dullness	Palpation [] no fremitus	Lymph nodes [] no axillary, inguinal, cervical or submandibular LAD
Anus/rectum [] no abnormality or masses [] heme negative stool	Ausculation [] CTA w/o W, R, or R	GU [] nl male/female exam
	Abnormals:	
Abnormals:		Psych [] nl cognition
CV Palpation [] PMI nondisplaced	**Neuro** Orientation [] AAO x 3	Abnormals:
Auscultation [] no murmur, gallop, or rub	Cranial nerves [] CN II-XII intact	
Carotids [] nl intensity w/o bruit	Sensory [] nl sensation	
JVD [] no jugulovenous distention	Reflexes [] 2+ & symmetrical	
Pulses [] 2+/= femoral & pedal pulses	Abnormals:	
Edema [] no pedal edema		
Abnormals		
Musculoskeletal Inspection ROM Strength Tone (✓ if normal) Abnormals:		**Other:**
Upper extremity [] [] [] [] Lower extremity [] [] [] []		
Gait [] nl gait and FROM		

Labs:

Assessment & Plan:

_____
_____
_____
_____
_____
_____
_____
_____
_____
_____
_____

Clinical Rotation_____   Date: _____

Chief Complaint:

_____

History of Present Illness:

_____
_____
_____
_____
_____

Review of Systems:

	Yes	No		Yes	No		Yes	No		Yes	No
General: fatigue	[]	[]	CV: chest pain	[]	[]	Bloody stool	[]	[]	Polydypsia	[]	[]
Weight loss	[]	[]	Edema	[]	[]	GU: dysuria	[]	[]	Polyphagia	[]	[]
Fever	[]	[]	PND	[]	[]	Frequency	[]	[]	Polyphagia	[]	[]
Chills	[]	[]	Orthopnea	[]	[]	Hematuria	[]	[]	Temp int	[]	[]
Night sweats	[]	[]	Palpitations	[]	[]	Discharge	[]	[]	Derm: rash	[]	[]
Eye: vision change	[]	[]	Claudication	[]	[]	Flank pain	[]	[]	Pruritis	[]	[]
Pain	[]	[]	Resp: cough	[]	[]	MS: arthralgia	[]	[]	Neuro: weakness	[]	[]
Redness	[]	[]	SOB	[]	[]	Arthritis	[]	[]	Seizures	[]	[]
ENT: headaches	[]	[]	Wheezing	[]	[]	Joint swelling	[]	[]	Parasthesias	[]	[]
Hoarseness	[]	[]	Hemoptysis	[]	[]	Myalgias	[]	[]	Tremors	[]	[]
Sore throat	[]	[]	GI: abd pain	[]	[]	Back pain	[]	[]	Syncope	[]	[]
Epistaxis	[]	[]	BM changes	[]	[]	Heme: bleeding	[]	[]	Psych: anxiety	[]	[]
Sinus Sx	[]	[]	N/V	[]	[]	Bruising	[]	[]	Depression	[]	[]
Hearing loss	[]	[]	Diarrhea	[]	[]	Lymph: swelling	[]	[]	Hallucinations	[]	[]
Tinnitus	[]	[]	Heartburn	[]	[]	Endo: polyuria	[]	[]	All/Imm: hayfever	[]	[]
									Runny nose	[]	[]

Other ROS: _____

Past Medical History:

_____
_____
_____
_____
_____
_____

Social History:

_____

Cigs: [] No Yes [] → Pack yrs _____
ETOH [] No Yes [] → Amount? _____
Illicits [] No Yes [] → Type?   _____
Allergies: [] NKDA _____
Medications:

_____

Past Surgical History:

_____
_____
_____
_____

_____
_____

Family History:

_____
_____
_____
_____

[] All other ROS reviewed and were NEGATIVE

Physical Exam T _____ BP _____ HR _____ Wt _____ (lbs) Ht _____ (in) BMI _____		
Eyes [] nl conjunctiva & lids	**ENT** External [] no scars, lesions, masses	**Neck** External [] no tracheal deviation
Pupils [] equal, round, & reactive	Otoscopic [] nl canals, TM	Palpation [] no masses
Fundus [] nl discs and vessels	Hearing [] nl hearing	Thyroid [] no enlargement
Vision [] acuity & gross fields intact	Oropharynx [] nl teeth, tongue, pharynx	Abnormals:
Abnormals:	Abnormals:	
GI Palpation [] no masses or tenderness [] no hep/splenomegaly	**Resp** Effort [] nl w/o retractions	**Skin** [] no rashes, or lesions
Ausculation [] nl bowel sounds	Percussion [] no dullness	Chest [] nl breast, no d/c
Percussion [] no dullness	Palpation [] no fremitus	Lymph nodes [] no axillary, inguinal, cervical or submandibular LAD
Anus/rectum [] no abnormality or masses [] heme negative stool	Ausculation [] CTA w/o W, R, or R	GU [] nl male/female exam
Abnormals:	Abnormals:	Psych [] nl cognition
CV Palpation [] PMI nondisplaced	**Neuro** Orientation [] AAO x 3	Abnormals:
Auscultation [] no murmur, gallop, or rub	Cranial nerves [] CN II-XII intact	
Carotids [] nl intensity w/o bruit	Sensory [] nl sensation	
JVD [] no jugulovenous distention	Reflexes [] 2+ & symmetrical	
Pulses [] 2+/= femoral & pedal pulses	Abnormals:	
Edema [] no pedal edema		
Abnormals		

Musculoskeletal	Inspection	ROM	Strength	Tone (✓ if normal)	Abnormals:	Other:
Upper extremity	[]	[]	[]	[]		
Lower extremity	[]	[]	[]	[]		
Gait	[] nl gait and FROM					

Labs:

Assessment & Plan:

_____
_____
_____
_____
_____
_____
_____
_____
_____
_____

Clinical Rotation_____   Date: _____

Chief Complaint:
_____

History of Present Illness:
_____
_____
_____
_____
_____

Review of Systems:

	Yes	No		Yes	No		Yes	No		Yes	No
General: fatigue	[]	[]	CV: chest pain	[]	[]	Bloody stool	[]	[]	Polydypsia	[]	[]
Weight loss	[]	[]	Edema	[]	[]	GU: dysuria	[]	[]	Polyphagia	[]	[]
Fever	[]	[]	PND	[]	[]	Frequency	[]	[]	Polyphagia	[]	[]
Chills	[]	[]	Orthopnea	[]	[]	Hematuria	[]	[]	Temp int	[]	[]
Night sweats	[]	[]	Palpitations	[]	[]	Discharge	[]	[]	Derm: rash	[]	[]
Eye: vision change	[]	[]	Claudication	[]	[]	Flank pain	[]	[]	Pruritis	[]	[]
Pain	[]	[]	Resp: cough	[]	[]	MS: arthralgia	[]	[]	Neuro: weakness	[]	[]
Redness	[]	[]	SOB	[]	[]	Arthritis	[]	[]	Seizures	[]	[]
ENT: headaches	[]	[]	Wheezing	[]	[]	Joint swelling	[]	[]	Parasthesias	[]	[]
Hoarseness	[]	[]	Hemoptysis	[]	[]	Myalgias	[]	[]	Tremors	[]	[]
Sore throat	[]	[]	GI: abd pain	[]	[]	Back pain	[]	[]	Syncope	[]	[]
Epistaxis	[]	[]	BM changes	[]	[]	Heme: bleeding	[]	[]	Psych: anxiety	[]	[]
Sinus Sx	[]	[]	N/V	[]	[]	Bruising	[]	[]	Depression	[]	[]
Hearing loss	[]	[]	Diarrhea	[]	[]	Lymph: swelling	[]	[]	Hallucinations	[]	[]
Tinnitus	[]	[]	Heartburn	[]	[]	Endo: polyuria	[]	[]	All/Imm: hayfever	[]	[]
									Runny nose	[]	[]

Other ROS: _____

Past Medical History:
_____
_____
_____
_____
_____
_____

Past Surgical History:
_____
_____
_____
_____

Family History:
_____
_____
_____

[] All other ROS reviewed and were NEGATIVE

Social History:
_____

Cigs: [] No Yes [] → Pack yrs _____
ETOH [] No Yes [] → Amount? _____
Illicits [] No Yes [] → Type? _____
Allergies: [] NKDA _____
Medications:
_____
_____
_____
_____
_____
_____
_____
_____
_____
_____

Physical Exam T _____ BP _____ HR _____ Wt _____ (lbs) Ht _____ (in) BMI _____

Eyes	[] nl conjunctiva & lids	**ENT** External [] no scars, lesions, masses	**Neck** External [] no tracheal deviation
Pupils	[] equal, round, & reactive	Otoscopic [] nl canals, TM	Palpation [] no masses
Fundus	[] nl discs and vessels	Hearing [] nl hearing	Thyroid [] no enlargement
Vision	[] acuity & gross fields intact	Oropharynx [] nl teeth, tongue, pharynx	Abnormals:
Abnormals:		Abnormals:	

GI Palpation [] no masses or tenderness [] no hep/splenomegaly	**Resp** Effort [] nl w/o retractions	**Skin** [] no rashes, or lesions
	Percussion [] no dullness	Chest [] nl breast, no d/c
Ausculation [] nl bowel sounds	Palpation [] no fremitus	Lymph nodes [] no axillary, inguinal, cervical or submandibular LAD
Percussion [] no dullness	Ausculation [] CTA w/o W, R, or R	
Anus/rectum [] no abnormality or masses [] heme negative stool	Abnormals:	GU [] nl male/female exam
Abnormals:		Psych [] nl cognition
CV Palpation [] PMI nondisplaced	**Neuro** Orientation [] AAO x 3	Abnormals:
Auscultation [] no murmur, gallop, or rub	Cranial nerves [] CN II-XII intact	
Carotids [] nl intensity w/o bruit	Sensory [] nl sensation	
JVD [] no jugulovenous distention	Reflexes [] 2+ & symmetrical	
Pulses [] 2+/= femoral & pedal pulses	Abnormals:	
Edema [] no pedal edema		
Abnormals		

Musculoskeletal	Inspection	ROM	Strength	Tone (✓ if normal)	Abnormals:	**Other:**
Upper extremity	[]	[]	[]	[]		
Lower extremity	[]	[]	[]	[]		
Gait	[] nl gait and FROM					

Labs:

Assessment & Plan:

_____
_____
_____
_____
_____
_____
_____
_____
_____
_____

Clinical Rotation_____   Date: _____

Chief Complaint:

_____

History of Present Illness:

_____
_____
_____
_____
_____
_____

Review of Systems:

	Yes	No		Yes	No		Yes	No		Yes	No
General: fatigue	[]	[]	CV: chest pain	[]	[]	Bloody stool	[]	[]	Polydypsia	[]	[]
Weight loss	[]	[]	Edema	[]	[]	GU: dysuria	[]	[]	Polyphagia	[]	[]
Fever	[]	[]	PND	[]	[]	Frequency	[]	[]	Polyphagia	[]	[]
Chills	[]	[]	Orthopnea	[]	[]	Hematuria	[]	[]	Temp int	[]	[]
Night sweats	[]	[]	Palpitations	[]	[]	Discharge	[]	[]	Derm: rash	[]	[]
Eye: vision change	[]	[]	Claudication	[]	[]	Flank pain	[]	[]	Pruritis	[]	[]
Pain	[]	[]	Resp: cough	[]	[]	MS: arthralgia	[]	[]	Neuro: weakness	[]	[]
Redness	[]	[]	SOB	[]	[]	Arthritis	[]	[]	Seizures	[]	[]
ENT: headaches	[]	[]	Wheezing	[]	[]	Joint swelling	[]	[]	Parasthesias	[]	[]
Hoarseness	[]	[]	Hemoptysis	[]	[]	Myalgias	[]	[]	Tremors	[]	[]
Sore throat	[]	[]	GI: abd pain	[]	[]	Back pain	[]	[]	Syncope	[]	[]
Epistaxis	[]	[]	BM changes	[]	[]	Heme: bleeding	[]	[]	Psych: anxiety	[]	[]
Sinus Sx	[]	[]	N/V	[]	[]	Bruising	[]	[]	Depression	[]	[]
Hearing loss	[]	[]	Diarrhea	[]	[]	Lymph: swelling	[]	[]	Hallucinations	[]	[]
Tinnitus	[]	[]	Heartburn	[]	[]	Endo: polyuria	[]	[]	All/Imm: hayfever	[]	[]
									Runny nose	[]	[]

Other ROS: _____

Past Medical History:

_____
_____
_____
_____
_____
_____

Past Surgical History:

_____
_____
_____
_____

Family History:

_____
_____
_____

[] All other ROS reviewed and were NEGATIVE

Social History:

_____

Cigs: [] No Yes [] → Pack yrs _____
ETOH [] No Yes [] → Amount? _____
Illicits [] No Yes [] → Type? _____
Allergies: [] NKDA _____
Medications:

_____
_____
_____
_____
_____
_____
_____
_____
_____
_____

Physical Exam   T _____   BP _____   HR _____   Wt _____(lbs)   Ht _____(in)   BMI _____

Eyes	[] nl conjunctiva & lids	**ENT** External	[] no scars, lesions, masses	**Neck** External	[] no tracheal deviation
Pupils	[] equal, round, & reactive	Otoscopic	[] nl canals, TM	Palpation	[] no masses
Fundus	[] nl discs and vessels	Hearing	[] nl hearing	Thyroid	[] no enlargement
Vision	[] acuity & gross fields intact	Oropharynx	[] nl teeth, tongue, pharynx	Abnormals:	
Abnormals:		Abnormals:			

GI Palpation []	no masses or tenderness	**Resp** Effort	[] nl w/o retractions	**Skin**	[] no rashes, or lesions
[]	no hep/splenomegaly	Percussion	[] no dullness	Chest	[] nl breast, no d/c
Ausculation []	nl bowel sounds	Palpation	[] no fremitus	Lymph nodes	[] no axillary, inguinal, cervical or submandibular LAD
Percussion []	no dullness	Ausculation	[] CTA w/o W, R, or R		
Anus/rectum []	no abnormality or masses	Abnormals:		GU	[] nl male/female exam
[]	heme negative stool				
Abnormals:				Psych	[] nl cognition

CV Palpation []	PMI nondisplaced	**Neuro** Orientation []	AAO x 3	Abnormals:	
Auscultation []	no murmur, gallop, or rub	Cranial nerves	[] CN II-XII intact		
Carotids []	nl intensity w/o bruit	Sensory	[] nl sensation		
JVD []	no jugulovenous distention	Reflexes	[] 2+ & symmetrical		
Pulses []	2+/= femoral & pedal pulses	Abnormals:			
Edema []	no pedal edema				
Abnormals					

Musculoskeletal	Inspection	ROM	Strength	Tone (✓ if normal)	Abnormals:	**Other:**
Upper extremity	[]	[]	[]	[]		
Lower extremity	[]	[]	[]	[]		
Gait	[] nl gait and FROM					

Labs:

Assessment & Plan:

_____
_____
_____
_____
_____
_____
_____
_____
_____
_____
_____

Clinical Rotation_____   Date: _____

Chief Complaint:

_____

History of Present Illness:

_____
_____
_____
_____
_____

Review of Systems:

	Yes	No		Yes	No		Yes	No		Yes	No
General: fatigue	[]	[]	CV: chest pain	[]	[]	Bloody stool	[]	[]	Polydipsia	[]	[]
Weight loss	[]	[]	Edema	[]	[]	GU: dysuria	[]	[]	Polyphagia	[]	[]
Fever	[]	[]	PND	[]	[]	Frequency	[]	[]	Polyphagia	[]	[]
Chills	[]	[]	Orthopnea	[]	[]	Hematuria	[]	[]	Temp int	[]	[]
Night sweats	[]	[]	Palpitations	[]	[]	Discharge	[]	[]	Derm: rash	[]	[]
Eye: vision change	[]	[]	Claudication	[]	[]	Flank pain	[]	[]	Pruritis	[]	[]
Pain	[]	[]	Resp: cough	[]	[]	MS: arthralgia	[]	[]	Neuro: weakness	[]	[]
Redness	[]	[]	SOB	[]	[]	Arthritis	[]	[]	Seizures	[]	[]
ENT: headaches	[]	[]	Wheezing	[]	[]	Joint swelling	[]	[]	Parasthesias	[]	[]
Hoarseness	[]	[]	Hemoptysis	[]	[]	Myalgias	[]	[]	Tremors	[]	[]
Sore throat	[]	[]	GI: abd pain	[]	[]	Back pain	[]	[]	Syncope	[]	[]
Epistaxis	[]	[]	BM changes	[]	[]	Heme: bleeding	[]	[]	Psych: anxiety	[]	[]
Sinus Sx	[]	[]	N/V	[]	[]	Bruising	[]	[]	Depression	[]	[]
Hearing loss	[]	[]	Diarrhea	[]	[]	Lymph: swelling	[]	[]	Hallucinations	[]	[]
Tinnitus	[]	[]	Heartburn	[]	[]	Endo: polyuria	[]	[]	All/Imm: hayfever	[]	[]
									Runny nose	[]	[]

Other ROS: _____

Past Medical History:

_____
_____
_____
_____
_____
_____

Past Surgical History:

_____
_____
_____
_____

Family History:

_____
_____
_____

[] All other ROS reviewed and were NEGATIVE

Social History:

_____

Cigs: [] No Yes [] → Pack yrs _____
ETOH [] No Yes [] → Amount? _____
Illicits [] No Yes [] → Type? _____
Allergies: [] NKDA _____
Medications:

_____
_____
_____
_____
_____
_____
_____
_____
_____

Physical Exam T _____	BP _____	HR _____	Wt _____(lbs)	Ht _____(in)	BMI _____

Eyes [] nl conjunctiva & lids	**ENT** External [] no scars, lesions, masses	**Neck** External [] no tracheal deviation
Pupils [] equal, round, & reactive	Otoscopic [] nl canals, TM	Palpation [] no masses
Fundus [] nl discs and vessels	Hearing [] nl hearing	Thyroid [] no enlargement
Vision [] acuity & gross fields intact	Oropharynx [] nl teeth, tongue, pharynx	Abnormals:
Abnormals:	Abnormals:	
GI Palpation [] no masses or tenderness [] no hep/splenomegaly	**Resp** Effort [] nl w/o retractions	**Skin** [] no rashes, or lesions
	Percussion [] no dullness	Chest [] nl breast, no d/c
Ausculation [] nl bowel sounds	Palpation [] no fremitus	Lymph nodes [] no axillary, inguinal, cervical or submandibular LAD
Percussion [] no dullness	Ausculation [] CTA w/o W, R, or R	
Anus/rectum [] no abnormality or masses [] heme negative stool	Abnormals:	GU [] nl male/female exam
Abnormals:		Psych [] nl cognition
CV Palpation [] PMI nondisplaced	**Neuro** Orientation [] AAO x 3	Abnormals:
Auscultation [] no murmur, gallop, or rub	Cranial nerves [] CN II-XII intact	
Carotids [] nl intensity w/o bruit	Sensory [] nl sensation	
JVD [] no jugulovenous distention	Reflexes [] 2+ & symmetrical	
Pulses [] 2+/= femoral & pedal pulses	Abnormals:	
Edema [] no pedal edema		
Abnormals		

Musculoskeletal Inspection ROM Strength Tone (✓ if normal) Abnormals:	**Other:**
Upper extremity [] [] [] [] Lower extremity [] [] [] []	
Gait [] nl gait and FROM	

Labs:

Assessment & Plan:

Clinical Rotation_____   Date: _____

Chief Complaint:
_____

History of Present Illness:
_____
_____
_____
_____
_____

Review of Systems:

	Yes	No		Yes	No		Yes	No		Yes	No
General: fatigue	[]	[]	CV: chest pain	[]	[]	Bloody stool	[]	[]	Polydypsia	[]	[]
Weight loss	[]	[]	Edema	[]	[]	GU: dysuria	[]	[]	Polyphagia	[]	[]
Fever	[]	[]	PND	[]	[]	Frequency	[]	[]	Polyphagia	[]	[]
Chills	[]	[]	Orthopnea	[]	[]	Hematuria	[]	[]	Temp int	[]	[]
Night sweats	[]	[]	Palpitations	[]	[]	Discharge	[]	[]	Derm: rash	[]	[]
Eye: vision change	[]	[]	Claudication	[]	[]	Flank pain	[]	[]	Pruritis	[]	[]
Pain	[]	[]	Resp: cough	[]	[]	MS: arthralgia	[]	[]	Neuro: weakness	[]	[]
Redness	[]	[]	SOB	[]	[]	Arthritis	[]	[]	Seizures	[]	[]
ENT: headaches	[]	[]	Wheezing	[]	[]	Joint swelling	[]	[]	Parasthesias	[]	[]
Hoarseness	[]	[]	Hemoptysis	[]	[]	Myalgias	[]	[]	Tremors	[]	[]
Sore throat	[]	[]	GI: abd pain	[]	[]	Back pain	[]	[]	Syncope	[]	[]
Epistaxis	[]	[]	BM changes	[]	[]	Heme: bleeding	[]	[]	Psych: anxiety	[]	[]
Sinus Sx	[]	[]	N/V	[]	[]	Bruising	[]	[]	Depression	[]	[]
Hearing loss	[]	[]	Diarrhea	[]	[]	Lymph: swelling	[]	[]	Hallucinations	[]	[]
Tinnitus	[]	[]	Heartburn	[]	[]	Endo: polyuria	[]	[]	All/Imm: hayfever	[]	[]
									Runny nose	[]	[]

Other ROS: _____

Past Medical History:
_____
_____
_____
_____
_____
_____
_____

Past Surgical History:
_____
_____
_____
_____

Family History:
_____
_____
_____

[ ] All other ROS reviewed and were NEGATIVE

Social History:
_____

Cigs: [] No Yes [] → Pack yrs _____
ETOH [] No Yes [] → Amount? _____
Illicits [] No Yes [] → Type?   _____
Allergies: [] NKDA _____
Medications:
_____
_____
_____
_____
_____
_____
_____
_____
_____
_____
_____
_____

Physical Exam   T _____   BP _____   HR _____   Wt _____ (lbs)   Ht _____ (in)   BMI _____

Eyes	[] nl conjunctiva & lids	ENT External	[] no scars, lesions, masses	Neck External	[] no tracheal deviation
Pupils	[] equal, round, & reactive	Otoscopic	[] nl canals, TM	Palpation	[] no masses
Fundus	[] nl discs and vessels	Hearing	[] nl hearing	Thyroid	[] no enlargement
Vision	[] acuity & gross fields intact	Oropharynx	[] nl teeth, tongue, pharynx	Abnormals:	
Abnormals:		Abnormals:			

GI Palpation [] no masses or tenderness [] no hep/splenomegaly	Resp Effort [] nl w/o retractions	Skin [] no rashes, or lesions
Ausculation [] nl bowel sounds	Percussion [] no dullness	Chest [] nl breast, no d/c
Percussion [] no dullness	Palpation [] no fremitus	Lymph nodes [] no axillary, inguinal, cervical or submandibular LAD
Anus/rectum [] no abnormality or masses [] heme negative stool	Ausculation [] CTA w/o W, R, or R	GU [] nl male/female exam
Abnormals:	Abnormals:	Psych [] nl cognition
CV Palpation [] PMI nondisplaced	Neuro Orientation [] AAO x 3	Abnormals:
Auscultation [] no murmur, gallop, or rub	Cranial nerves [] CN II-XII intact	
Carotids [] nl intensity w/o bruit	Sensory [] nl sensation	
JVD [] no jugulovenous distention	Reflexes [] 2+ & symmetrical	
Pulses [] 2+/= femoral & pedal pulses	Abnormals:	
Edema [] no pedal edema		
Abnormals		

Musculoskeletal	Inspection	ROM	Strength	Tone (✓ if normal)	Abnormals:	Other:
Upper extremity	[]	[]	[]	[]		
Lower extremity	[]	[]	[]	[]		
Gait	[] nl gait and FROM					

Labs:

Assessment & Plan:

_____
_____
_____
_____
_____
_____
_____
_____
_____
_____

Clinical Rotation_____   Date: _____

Chief Complaint:

History of Present Illness:

Review of Systems:

	Yes	No		Yes	No		Yes	No		Yes	No
General: fatigue	[]	[]	CV: chest pain	[]	[]	Bloody stool	[]	[]	Polydypsia	[]	[]
Weight loss	[]	[]	Edema	[]	[]	GU: dysuria	[]	[]	Polyphagia	[]	[]
Fever	[]	[]	PND	[]	[]	Frequency	[]	[]	Polyphagia	[]	[]
Chills	[]	[]	Orthopnea	[]	[]	Hematuria	[]	[]	Temp int	[]	[]
Night sweats	[]	[]	Palpitations	[]	[]	Discharge	[]	[]	Derm: rash	[]	[]
Eye: vision change	[]	[]	Claudication	[]	[]	Flank pain	[]	[]	Pruritis	[]	[]
Pain	[]	[]	Resp: cough	[]	[]	MS: arthralgia	[]	[]	Neuro: weakness	[]	[]
Redness	[]	[]	SOB	[]	[]	Arthritis	[]	[]	Seizures	[]	[]
ENT: headaches	[]	[]	Wheezing	[]	[]	Joint swelling	[]	[]	Parasthesias	[]	[]
Hoarseness	[]	[]	Hemoptysis	[]	[]	Myalgias	[]	[]	Tremors	[]	[]
Sore throat	[]	[]	GI: abd pain	[]	[]	Back pain	[]	[]	Syncope	[]	[]
Epistaxis	[]	[]	BM changes	[]	[]	Heme: bleeding	[]	[]	Psych: anxiety	[]	[]
Sinus Sx	[]	[]	N/V	[]	[]	Bruising	[]	[]	Depression	[]	[]
Hearing loss	[]	[]	Diarrhea	[]	[]	Lymph: swelling	[]	[]	Hallucinations	[]	[]
Tinnitus	[]	[]	Heartburn	[]	[]	Endo: polyuria	[]	[]	All/Imm: hayfever	[]	[]
									Runny nose	[]	[]

Other ROS: _____

Past Medical History:

Social History:

Cigs: [] No Yes [] → Pack yrs _____
ETOH [] No Yes [] → Amount? _____
Illicits [] No Yes [] → Type? _____
Allergies: [] NKDA _____
Medications:

Past Surgical History:

Family History:

[] All other ROS reviewed and were NEGATIVE

Physical Exam	T _____	BP _____	HR _____	Wt _____ (lbs)	Ht _____ (in)	BMI _____

Eyes	[] nl conjunctiva & lids	ENT External	[] no scars, lesions, masses	Neck External	[] no tracheal deviation
Pupils	[] equal, round, & reactive	Otoscopic	[] nl canals, TM	Palpation	[] no masses
Fundus	[] nl discs and vessels	Hearing	[] nl hearing	Thyroid	[] no enlargement
Vision	[] acuity & gross fields intact	Oropharynx	[] nl teeth, tongue, pharynx	Abnormals:	
Abnormals:		Abnormals:			

GI Palpation	[] no masses or tenderness [] no hep/splenomegaly	Resp Effort	[] nl w/o retractions	Skin	[] no rashes, or lesions
Ausculation	[] nl bowel sounds	Percussion	[] no dullness	Chest	[] nl breast, no d/c
Percussion	[] no dullness	Palpation	[] no fremitus	Lymph nodes	[] no axillary, inguinal, cervical or submandibular LAD
Anus/rectum	[] no abnormality or masses [] heme negative stool	Ausculation	[] CTA w/o W, R, or R	GU	[] nl male/female exam
Abnormals:		Abnormals:		Psych	[] nl cognition

CV Palpation	[] PMI nondisplaced	Neuro Orientation	[] AAO x 3	Abnormals:
Auscultation	[] no murmur, gallop, or rub	Cranial nerves	[] CN II-XII intact	
Carotids	[] nl intensity w/o bruit	Sensory	[] nl sensation	
JVD	[] no jugulovenous distention	Reflexes	[] 2+ & symmetrical	
Pulses	[] 2+/= femoral & pedal pulses	Abnormals:		
Edema	[] no pedal edema			
Abnormals				

Musculoskeletal	Inspection	ROM	Strength	Tone	(✓ if normal)	Abnormals:	Other:
Upper extremity	[]	[]	[]	[]			
Lower extremity	[]	[]	[]	[]			
Gait	[] nl gait and FROM						

Labs:

Assessment & Plan:

_____
_____
_____
_____
_____
_____
_____
_____
_____
_____
_____
_____

Clinical Rotation_____   Date: _____

Chief Complaint:

_____

History of Present Illness:

_____
_____
_____
_____
_____
_____

Review of Systems:

	Yes No		Yes No		Yes No		Yes No
General: fatigue	[] []	CV: chest pain	[] []	Bloody stool	[] []	Polydypsia	[] []
Weight loss	[] []	Edema	[] []	GU: dysuria	[] []	Polyphagia	[] []
Fever	[] []	PND	[] []	Frequency	[] []	Polyphagia	[] []
Chills	[] []	Orthopnea	[] []	Hematuria	[] []	Temp int	[] []
Night sweats	[] []	Palpitations	[] []	Discharge	[] []	Derm: rash	[] []
Eye: vision change	[] []	Claudication	[] []	Flank pain	[] []	Pruritis	[] []
Pain	[] []	Resp: cough	[] []	MS: arthralgia	[] []	Neuro: weakness	[] []
Redness	[] []	SOB	[] []	Arthritis	[] []	Seizures	[] []
ENT: headaches	[] []	Wheezing	[] []	Joint swelling	[] []	Parasthesias	[] []
Hoarseness	[] []	Hemoptysis	[] []	Myalgias	[] []	Tremors	[] []
Sore throat	[] []	GI: abd pain	[] []	Back pain	[] []	Syncope	[] []
Epistaxis	[] []	BM changes	[] []	Heme: bleeding	[] []	Psych: anxiety	[] []
Sinus Sx	[] []	N/V	[] []	Bruising	[] []	Depression	[] []
Hearing loss	[] []	Diarrhea	[] []	Lymph: swelling	[] []	Hallucinations	[] []
Tinnitus	[] []	Heartburn	[] []	Endo: polyuria	[] []	All/Imm: hayfever	[] []
						Runny nose	[] []

Other ROS: _____

Past Medical History:

_____
_____
_____
_____
_____
_____

Past Surgical History:

_____
_____
_____
_____

Family History:

_____
_____

Social History:

_____

Cigs: [] No Yes [] → Pack yrs _____
ETOH [] No Yes [] → Amount? _____
Illicits [] No Yes [] → Type? _____
Allergies: [] NKDA _____
Medications:

_____
_____
_____
_____
_____
_____
_____
_____

[] All other ROS reviewed and were NEGATIVE

Physical Exam T _____ BP _____	HR _____ Wt ____(lbs)	Ht ____(in) BMI _____
Eyes [] nl conjunctiva & lids	**ENT** External [] no scars, lesions, masses	**Neck** External [] no tracheal deviation
Pupils [] equal, round, & reactive	Otoscopic [] nl canals, TM	Palpation [] no masses
Fundus [] nl discs and vessels	Hearing [] nl hearing	Thyroid [] no enlargement
Vision [] acuity & gross fields intact	Oropharynx [] nl teeth, tongue, pharynx	Abnormals:
Abnormals:	Abnormals:	
GI Palpation [] no masses or tenderness [] no hep/splenomegaly	**Resp** Effort [] nl w/o retractions	**Skin** [] no rashes, or lesions
Ausculation [] nl bowel sounds	Percussion [] no dullness	Chest [] nl breast, no d/c
Percussion [] no dullness	Palpation [] no fremitus	Lymph nodes [] no axillary, inguinal, cervical or submandibular LAD
Anus/rectum [] no abnormality or masses [] heme negative stool	Ausculation [] CTA w/o W, R, or R	GU [] nl male/female exam
Abnormals:	Abnormals:	Psych [] nl cognition
CV Palpation [] PMI nondisplaced	**Neuro** Orientation [] AAO x 3	Abnormals:
Auscultation [] no murmur, gallop, or rub	Cranial nerves [] CN II-XII intact	
Carotids [] nl intensity w/o bruit	Sensory [] nl sensation	
JVD [] no jugulovenous distention	Reflexes [] 2+ & symmetrical	
Pulses [] 2+/= femoral & pedal pulses	Abnormals:	
Edema [] no pedal edema		
Abnormals		

Musculoskeletal Inspection ROM Strength Tone (✓ if normal) Abnormals:	**Other:**
Upper extremity [] [] [] [] Lower extremity [] [] [] []	
Gait [] nl gait and FROM	

Labs:

Assessment & Plan:

_____
_____
_____
_____
_____
_____
_____
_____
_____
_____
_____

Clinical Rotation_____   Date: _____

Chief Complaint:
_____

History of Present Illness:
_____
_____
_____
_____
_____

Review of Systems:

	Yes	No		Yes	No		Yes	No		Yes	No
General: fatigue	[]	[]	CV: chest pain	[]	[]	Bloody stool	[]	[]	Polydypsia	[]	[]
Weight loss	[]	[]	Edema	[]	[]	GU: dysuria	[]	[]	Polyphagia	[]	[]
Fever	[]	[]	PND	[]	[]	Frequency	[]	[]	Polyphagia	[]	[]
Chills	[]	[]	Orthopnea	[]	[]	Hematuria	[]	[]	Temp int	[]	[]
Night sweats	[]	[]	Palpitations	[]	[]	Discharge	[]	[]	Derm: rash	[]	[]
Eye: vision change	[]	[]	Claudication	[]	[]	Flank pain	[]	[]	Pruritis	[]	[]
Pain	[]	[]	Resp: cough	[]	[]	MS: arthralgia	[]	[]	Neuro: weakness	[]	[]
Redness	[]	[]	SOB	[]	[]	Arthritis	[]	[]	Seizures	[]	[]
ENT: headaches	[]	[]	Wheezing	[]	[]	Joint swelling	[]	[]	Parasthesias	[]	[]
Hoarseness	[]	[]	Hemoptysis	[]	[]	Myalgias	[]	[]	Tremors	[]	[]
Sore throat	[]	[]	GI: abd pain	[]	[]	Back pain	[]	[]	Syncope	[]	[]
Epistaxis	[]	[]	BM changes	[]	[]	Heme: bleeding	[]	[]	Psych: anxiety	[]	[]
Sinus Sx	[]	[]	N/V	[]	[]	Bruising	[]	[]	Depression	[]	[]
Hearing loss	[]	[]	Diarrhea	[]	[]	Lymph: swelling	[]	[]	Hallucinations	[]	[]
Tinnitus	[]	[]	Heartburn	[]	[]	Endo: polyuria	[]	[]	All/Imm: hayfever	[]	[]
									Runny nose	[]	[]

Other ROS: _____

Past Medical History:
_____
_____
_____
_____
_____
_____
_____

Past Surgical History:
_____
_____
_____
_____

Family History:
_____
_____
_____
_____

[] All other ROS reviewed and were NEGATIVE

Social History:
_____

Cigs: [] No Yes [] → Pack yrs _____
ETOH [] No Yes [] → Amount? _____
Illicits [] No Yes [] → Type? _____
Allergies: [] NKDA _____
Medications:
_____
_____
_____
_____
_____
_____
_____
_____
_____
_____
_____
_____

Physical Exam T _____	BP _____	HR _____	Wt _____(lbs)	Ht _____(in)	BMI _____

Eyes [] nl conjunctiva & lids	**ENT** External [] no scars, lesions, masses	**Neck** External [] no tracheal deviation
Pupils [] equal, round, & reactive	Otoscopic [] nl canals, TM	Palpation [] no masses
Fundus [] nl discs and vessels	Hearing [] nl hearing	Thyroid [] no enlargement
Vision [] acuity & gross fields intact	Oropharynx [] nl teeth, tongue, pharynx	Abnormals:
Abnormals:	Abnormals:	
GI Palpation [] no masses or tenderness [] no hep/splenomegaly	**Resp** Effort [] nl w/o retractions	**Skin** [] no rashes, or lesions
	Percussion [] no dullness	Chest [] nl breast, no d/c
Ausculation [] nl bowel sounds	Palpation [] no fremitus	Lymph nodes [] no axillary, inguinal, cervical or submandibular LAD
Percussion [] no dullness	Ausculation [] CTA w/o W, R, or R	
Anus/rectum [] no abnormality or masses [] heme negative stool	Abnormals:	GU [] nl male/female exam
Abnormals:		Psych [] nl cognition
CV Palpation [] PMI nondisplaced	**Neuro** Orientation [] AAO x 3	Abnormals:
Auscultation [] no murmur, gallop, or rub	Cranial nerves [] CN II-XII intact	
Carotids [] nl intensity w/o bruit	Sensory [] nl sensation	
JVD [] no jugulovenous distention	Reflexes [] 2+ & symmetrical	
Pulses [] 2+/= femoral & pedal pulses	Abnormals:	
Edema [] no pedal edema		
Abnormals		

Musculoskeletal Inspection ROM Strength Tone (✓ if normal) Abnormals:	**Other:**
Upper extremity [] [] [] [] Lower extremity [] [] [] []	
Gait [] nl gait and FROM	

Labs:

Assessment & Plan:
_____
_____
_____
_____
_____
_____
_____
_____
_____
_____
_____

Clinical Rotation_____   Date: _____

Chief Complaint:
_____

History of Present Illness:
_____
_____
_____
_____
_____

Review of Systems:

	Yes	No		Yes	No		Yes	No		Yes	No
General: fatigue	[]	[]	CV: chest pain	[]	[]	Bloody stool	[]	[]	Polydypsia	[]	[]
Weight loss	[]	[]	Edema	[]	[]	GU: dysuria	[]	[]	Polyphagia	[]	[]
Fever	[]	[]	PND	[]	[]	Frequency	[]	[]	Polyphagia	[]	[]
Chills	[]	[]	Orthopnea	[]	[]	Hematuria	[]	[]	Temp int	[]	[]
Night sweats	[]	[]	Palpitations	[]	[]	Discharge	[]	[]	Derm: rash	[]	[]
Eye: vision change	[]	[]	Claudication	[]	[]	Flank pain	[]	[]	Pruritis	[]	[]
Pain	[]	[]	Resp: cough	[]	[]	MS: arthralgia	[]	[]	Neuro: weakness	[]	[]
Redness	[]	[]	SOB	[]	[]	Arthritis	[]	[]	Seizures	[]	[]
ENT: headaches	[]	[]	Wheezing	[]	[]	Joint swelling	[]	[]	Parasthesias	[]	[]
Hoarseness	[]	[]	Hemoptysis	[]	[]	Myalgias	[]	[]	Tremors	[]	[]
Sore throat	[]	[]	GI: abd pain	[]	[]	Back pain	[]	[]	Syncope	[]	[]
Epistaxis	[]	[]	BM changes	[]	[]	Heme: bleeding	[]	[]	Psych: anxiety	[]	[]
Sinus Sx	[]	[]	N/V	[]	[]	Bruising	[]	[]	Depression	[]	[]
Hearing loss	[]	[]	Diarrhea	[]	[]	Lymph: swelling	[]	[]	Hallucinations	[]	[]
Tinnitus	[]	[]	Heartburn	[]	[]	Endo: polyuria	[]	[]	All/Imm: hayfever	[]	[]
									Runny nose	[]	[]

Other ROS: _____

Past Medical History:
_____
_____
_____
_____
_____
_____
_____

Past Surgical History:
_____
_____
_____
_____

Family History:
_____
_____
_____

[] All other ROS reviewed and were NEGATIVE

Social History:
_____

Cigs: [] No Yes [] → Pack yrs _____
ETOH [] No Yes [] → Amount? _____
Illicits [] No Yes [] → Type? _____
Allergies: [] NKDA _____
Medications:
_____
_____
_____
_____
_____
_____
_____
_____
_____

Physical Exam T _____ BP _____ HR _____ Wt _____ (lbs) Ht _____ (in) BMI _____		
Eyes [] nl conjunctiva & lids	**ENT** External [] no scars, lesions, masses	**Neck** External [] no tracheal deviation
Pupils [] equal, round, & reactive	Otoscopic [] nl canals, TM	Palpation [] no masses
Fundus [] nl discs and vessels	Hearing [] nl hearing	Thyroid [] no enlargement
Vision [] acuity & gross fields intact	Oropharynx [] nl teeth, tongue, pharynx	Abnormals:
Abnormals:	Abnormals:	
GI Palpation [] no masses or tenderness [] no hep/splenomegaly	**Resp** Effort [] nl w/o retractions	**Skin** [] no rashes, or lesions
	Percussion [] no dullness	Chest [] nl breast, no d/c
Ausculation [] nl bowel sounds	Palpation [] no fremitus	Lymph nodes [] no axillary, inguinal, cervical or submandibular LAD
Percussion [] no dullness	Ausculation [] CTA w/o W, R, or R	
Anus/rectum [] no abnormality or masses [] heme negative stool	Abnormals:	GU [] nl male/female exam
Abnormals:		Psych [] nl cognition
CV Palpation [] PMI nondisplaced	**Neuro** Orientation [] AAO x 3	Abnormals:
Auscultation [] no murmur, gallop, or rub	Cranial nerves [] CN II-XII intact	
Carotids [] nl intensity w/o bruit	Sensory [] nl sensation	
JVD [] no jugulovenous distention	Reflexes [] 2+ & symmetrical	
Pulses [] 2+/= femoral & pedal pulses	Abnormals:	
Edema [] no pedal edema		
Abnormals		

Musculoskeletal	Inspection	ROM	Strength	Tone (✓ if normal)	Abnormals:	**Other:**
Upper extremity	[]	[]	[]	[]		
Lower extremity	[]	[]	[]	[]		
Gait [] nl gait and FROM						

Labs:

Assessment & Plan:
_____
_____
_____
_____
_____
_____
_____
_____
_____
_____
_____

Clinical Rotation_____   Date: _____

Chief Complaint:
_____

History of Present Illness:
_____
_____
_____
_____
_____

Review of Systems:

	Yes	No		Yes	No		Yes	No		Yes	No
General: fatigue	[]	[]	CV: chest pain	[]	[]	Bloody stool	[]	[]	Polydypsia	[]	[]
Weight loss	[]	[]	Edema	[]	[]	GU: dysuria	[]	[]	Polyphagia	[]	[]
Fever	[]	[]	PND	[]	[]	Frequency	[]	[]	Polyphagia	[]	[]
Chills	[]	[]	Orthopnea	[]	[]	Hematuria	[]	[]	Temp int	[]	[]
Night sweats	[]	[]	Palpitations	[]	[]	Discharge	[]	[]	Derm: rash	[]	[]
Eye: vision change	[]	[]	Claudication	[]	[]	Flank pain	[]	[]	Pruritis	[]	[]
Pain	[]	[]	Resp: cough	[]	[]	MS: arthralgia	[]	[]	Neuro: weakness	[]	[]
Redness	[]	[]	SOB	[]	[]	Arthritis	[]	[]	Seizures	[]	[]
ENT: headaches	[]	[]	Wheezing	[]	[]	Joint swelling	[]	[]	Parasthesias	[]	[]
Hoarseness	[]	[]	Hemoptysis	[]	[]	Myalgias	[]	[]	Tremors	[]	[]
Sore throat	[]	[]	GI: abd pain	[]	[]	Back pain	[]	[]	Syncope	[]	[]
Epistaxis	[]	[]	BM changes	[]	[]	Heme: bleeding	[]	[]	Psych: anxiety	[]	[]
Sinus Sx	[]	[]	N/V	[]	[]	Bruising	[]	[]	Depression	[]	[]
Hearing loss	[]	[]	Diarrhea	[]	[]	Lymph: swelling	[]	[]	Hallucinations	[]	[]
Tinnitus	[]	[]	Heartburn	[]	[]	Endo: polyuria	[]	[]	All/Imm: hayfever	[]	[]
									Runny nose	[]	[]

Other ROS: _____

Past Medical History:
_____
_____
_____
_____
_____
_____

Past Surgical History:
_____
_____
_____

Family History:
_____
_____

[] All other ROS reviewed and were NEGATIVE

Social History:
_____

Cigs: [] No Yes [] → Pack yrs _____
ETOH [] No Yes [] → Amount? _____
Illicits [] No Yes [] → Type?   _____
Allergies: [] NKDA _____
Medications:
_____
_____
_____
_____
_____
_____
_____
_____
_____

Physical Exam T _____ BP _____ HR _____ Wt _____(lbs) Ht _____(in) BMI _____

Eyes		**ENT** External		**Neck** External	
Eyes	[] nl conjunctiva & lids	ENT External	[] no scars, lesions, masses	Neck External	[] no tracheal deviation
Pupils	[] equal, round, & reactive	Otoscopic	[] nl canals, TM	Palpation	[] no masses
Fundus	[] nl discs and vessels	Hearing	[] nl hearing	Thyroid	[] no enlargement
Vision	[] acuity & gross fields intact	Oropharynx	[] nl teeth, tongue, pharynx	Abnormals:	
Abnormals:		Abnormals:			

GI Palpation	[] no masses or tenderness [] no hep/splenomegaly	**Resp** Effort	[] nl w/o retractions	**Skin**	[] no rashes, or lesions
Ausculation	[] nl bowel sounds	Percussion	[] no dullness	Chest	[] nl breast, no d/c
Percussion	[] no dullness	Palpation	[] no fremitus	Lymph nodes	[] no axillary, inguinal, cervical or submandibular LAD
Anus/rectum	[] no abnormality or masses [] heme negative stool	Ausculation	[] CTA w/o W, R, or R	GU	[] nl male/female exam
Abnormals:		Abnormals:		Psych	[] nl cognition

CV Palpation	[] PMI nondisplaced	**Neuro** Orientation	[] AAO x 3	Abnormals:	
Auscultation	[] no murmur, gallop, or rub	Cranial nerves	[] CN II-XII intact		
Carotids	[] nl intensity w/o bruit	Sensory	[] nl sensation		
JVD	[] no jugulovenous distention	Reflexes	[] 2+ & symmetrical		
Pulses	[] 2+/= femoral & pedal pulses	Abnormals:			
Edema	[] no pedal edema				
Abnormals					

Musculoskeletal	Inspection	ROM	Strength	Tone (✓ if normal)	Abnormals:	**Other:**
Upper extremity	[]	[]	[]	[]		
Lower extremity	[]	[]	[]	[]		
Gait	[] nl gait and FROM					

Labs:

Assessment & Plan:

Clinical Rotation_____   Date: _____

Chief Complaint:
_____

History of Present Illness:
_____
_____
_____
_____
_____
_____

Review of Systems:

	Yes	No		Yes	No		Yes	No		Yes	No
General: fatigue	☐	☐	CV: chest pain	☐	☐	Bloody stool	☐	☐	Polydypsia	☐	☐
Weight loss	☐	☐	Edema	☐	☐	GU: dysuria	☐	☐	Polyphagia	☐	☐
Fever	☐	☐	PND	☐	☐	Frequency	☐	☐	Polyphagia	☐	☐
Chills	☐	☐	Orthopnea	☐	☐	Hematuria	☐	☐	Temp int	☐	☐
Night sweats	☐	☐	Palpitations	☐	☐	Discharge	☐	☐	Derm: rash	☐	☐
Eye: vision change	☐	☐	Claudication	☐	☐	Flank pain	☐	☐	Pruritis	☐	☐
Pain	☐	☐	Resp: cough	☐	☐	MS: arthralgia	☐	☐	Neuro: weakness	☐	☐
Redness	☐	☐	SOB	☐	☐	Arthritis	☐	☐	Seizures	☐	☐
ENT: headaches	☐	☐	Wheezing	☐	☐	Joint swelling	☐	☐	Parasthesias	☐	☐
Hoarseness	☐	☐	Hemoptysis	☐	☐	Myalgias	☐	☐	Tremors	☐	☐
Sore throat	☐	☐	GI: abd pain	☐	☐	Back pain	☐	☐	Syncope	☐	☐
Epistaxis	☐	☐	BM changes	☐	☐	Heme: bleeding	☐	☐	Psych: anxiety	☐	☐
Sinus Sx	☐	☐	N/V	☐	☐	Bruising	☐	☐	Depression	☐	☐
Hearing loss	☐	☐	Diarrhea	☐	☐	Lymph: swelling	☐	☐	Hallucinations	☐	☐
Tinnitus	☐	☐	Heartburn	☐	☐	Endo: polyuria	☐	☐	All/Imm: hayfever	☐	☐
									Runny nose	☐	☐

Other ROS: _____

Past Medical History:
_____
_____
_____
_____
_____
_____
_____

Past Surgical History:
_____
_____
_____
_____

Family History:
_____
_____

[] All other ROS reviewed and were NEGATIVE

Social History:
_____

Cigs: ☐ No Yes ☐ → Pack yrs _____
ETOH ☐ No Yes ☐ → Amount? _____
Illicits ☐ No Yes ☐ → Type? _____
Allergies: ☐ NKDA _____
Medications:
_____
_____
_____
_____
_____
_____
_____
_____
_____

Physical Exam   T _____   BP _____   HR _____   Wt _____(lbs)   Ht _____(in)   BMI _____

Eyes	[] nl conjunctiva & lids	**ENT** External	[] no scars, lesions, masses	**Neck** External	[] no tracheal deviation
Pupils	[] equal, round, & reactive	Otoscopic	[] nl canals, TM	Palpation	[] no masses
Fundus	[] nl discs and vessels	Hearing	[] nl hearing	Thyroid	[] no enlargement
Vision	[] acuity & gross fields intact	Oropharynx	[] nl teeth, tongue, pharynx	Abnormals:	
Abnormals:		Abnormals:			

GI Palpation	[] no masses or tenderness [] no hep/splenomegaly	**Resp** Effort	[] nl w/o retractions	**Skin**	[] no rashes, or lesions
		Percussion	[] no dullness	Chest	[] nl breast, no d/c
Ausculation	[] nl bowel sounds	Palpation	[] no fremitus	Lymph nodes	[] no axillary, inguinal, cervical or submandibular LAD
Percussion	[] no dullness	Ausculation	[] CTA w/o W, R, or R		
Anus/rectum	[] no abnormality or masses [] heme negative stool	Abnormals:		GU	[] nl male/female exam
Abnormals:				Psych	[] nl cognition

CV Palpation	[] PMI nondisplaced	**Neuro** Orientation	[] AAO x 3	Abnormals:	
Auscultation	[] no murmur, gallop, or rub	Cranial nerves	[] CN II-XII intact		
Carotids	[] nl intensity w/o bruit	Sensory	[] nl sensation		
JVD	[] no jugulovenous distention	Reflexes	[] 2+ & symmetrical		
Pulses	[] 2+/= femoral & pedal pulses	Abnormals:			
Edema	[] no pedal edema				
Abnormals					

Musculoskeletal	Inspection	ROM	Strength	Tone (✓ if normal)	Abnormals:	**Other:**
Upper extremity	[]	[]	[]	[]		
Lower extremity	[]	[]	[]	[]		
Gait	[] nl gait and FROM					

Labs:

Assessment & Plan:

_____
_____
_____
_____
_____
_____
_____
_____
_____
_____
_____

Clinical Rotation_____   Date: _____

Chief Complaint:
_____

History of Present Illness:
_____
_____
_____
_____
_____

Review of Systems:

	Yes	No		Yes	No		Yes	No		Yes	No
General: fatigue	[]	[]	CV: chest pain	[]	[]	Bloody stool	[]	[]	Polydypsia	[]	[]
Weight loss	[]	[]	Edema	[]	[]	GU: dysuria	[]	[]	Polyphagia	[]	[]
Fever	[]	[]	PND	[]	[]	Frequency	[]	[]	Polyphagia	[]	[]
Chills	[]	[]	Orthopnea	[]	[]	Hematuria	[]	[]	Temp int	[]	[]
Night sweats	[]	[]	Palpitations	[]	[]	Discharge	[]	[]	Derm: rash	[]	[]
Eye: vision change	[]	[]	Claudication	[]	[]	Flank pain	[]	[]	Pruritis	[]	[]
Pain	[]	[]	Resp: cough	[]	[]	MS: arthralgia	[]	[]	Neuro: weakness	[]	[]
Redness	[]	[]	SOB	[]	[]	Arthritis	[]	[]	Seizures	[]	[]
ENT: headaches	[]	[]	Wheezing	[]	[]	Joint swelling	[]	[]	Parasthesias	[]	[]
Hoarseness	[]	[]	Hemoptysis	[]	[]	Myalgias	[]	[]	Tremors	[]	[]
Sore throat	[]	[]	GI: abd pain	[]	[]	Back pain	[]	[]	Syncope	[]	[]
Epistaxis	[]	[]	BM changes	[]	[]	Heme: bleeding	[]	[]	Psych: anxiety	[]	[]
Sinus Sx	[]	[]	N/V	[]	[]	Bruising	[]	[]	Depression	[]	[]
Hearing loss	[]	[]	Diarrhea	[]	[]	Lymph: swelling	[]	[]	Hallucinations	[]	[]
Tinnitus	[]	[]	Heartburn	[]	[]	Endo: polyuria	[]	[]	All/Imm: hayfever	[]	[]
									Runny nose	[]	[]

Other ROS:
_____

Past Medical History:
_____
_____
_____
_____
_____
_____
_____

Past Surgical History:
_____
_____
_____
_____

Family History:
_____
_____
_____

[] All other ROS reviewed and were NEGATIVE

Social History:
_____

Cigs: [] No Yes [] → Pack yrs _____
ETOH [] No Yes [] → Amount? _____
Illicits [] No Yes [] → Type? _____
Allergies: [] NKDA _____
Medications:
_____
_____
_____
_____
_____
_____
_____

Physical Exam T _____ BP _____ HR _____ Wt _____ (lbs) Ht _____ (in) BMI _____

Eyes		ENT External	[] no scars, lesions, masses	Neck External	[] no tracheal deviation
Eyes	[] nl conjunctiva & lids	ENT External	[] no scars, lesions, masses	Neck External	[] no tracheal deviation
Pupils	[] equal, round, & reactive	Otoscopic	[] nl canals, TM	Palpation	[] no masses
Fundus	[] nl discs and vessels	Hearing	[] nl hearing	Thyroid	[] no enlargement
Vision	[] acuity & gross fields intact	Oropharynx	[] nl teeth, tongue, pharynx	Abnormals:	
Abnormals:		Abnormals:			

GI Palpation	[] no masses or tenderness [] no hep/splenomegaly	Resp Effort	[] nl w/o retractions	Skin	[] no rashes, or lesions
Ausculation	[] nl bowel sounds	Percussion	[] no dullness	Chest	[] nl breast, no d/c
Percussion	[] no dullness	Palpation	[] no fremitus	Lymph nodes	[] no axillary, inguinal, cervical or submandibular LAD
Anus/rectum	[] no abnormality or masses [] heme negative stool	Ausculation	[] CTA w/o W, R, or R	GU	[] nl male/female exam
Abnormals:		Abnormals:		Psych	[] nl cognition

CV Palpation	[] PMI nondisplaced	Neuro Orientation	[] AAO x 3	Abnormals:	
Auscultation	[] no murmur, gallop, or rub	Cranial nerves	[] CN II-XII intact		
Carotids	[] nl intensity w/o bruit	Sensory	[] nl sensation		
JVD	[] no jugulovenous distention	Reflexes	[] 2+ & symmetrical		
Pulses	[] 2+/= femoral & pedal pulses	Abnormals:			
Edema	[] no pedal edema				
Abnormals					

Musculoskeletal Inspection ROM Strength Tone (✓ if normal)   Abnormals: **Other:**

	Inspection	ROM	Strength	Tone
Upper extremity	[]	[]	[]	[]
Lower extremity	[]	[]	[]	[]

Gait   []   nl gait and FROM

Labs:

Assessment & Plan:

Clinical Rotation_____   Date: _____

Chief Complaint:
_____

History of Present Illness:
_____
_____
_____
_____
_____

Review of Systems:

	Yes No		Yes No		Yes No		Yes No
General: fatigue	[] []	CV: chest pain	[] []	Bloody stool	[] []	Polydypsia	[] []
Weight loss	[] []	Edema	[] []	GU: dysuria	[] []	Polyphagia	[] []
Fever	[] []	PND	[] []	Frequency	[] []	Polyphagia	[] []
Chills	[] []	Orthopnea	[] []	Hematuria	[] []	Temp int	[] []
Night sweats	[] []	Palpitations	[] []	Discharge	[] []	Derm: rash	[] []
Eye: vision change	[] []	Claudication	[] []	Flank pain	[] []	Pruritis	[] []
Pain	[] []	Resp: cough	[] []	MS: arthralgia	[] []	Neuro: weakness	[] []
Redness	[] []	SOB	[] []	Arthritis	[] []	Seizures	[] []
ENT: headaches	[] []	Wheezing	[] []	Joint swelling	[] []	Parasthesias	[] []
Hoarseness	[] []	Hemoptysis	[] []	Myalgias	[] []	Tremors	[] []
Sore throat	[] []	GI: abd pain	[] []	Back pain	[] []	Syncope	[] []
Epistaxis	[] []	BM changes	[] []	Heme: bleeding	[] []	Psych: anxiety	[] []
Sinus Sx	[] []	N/V	[] []	Bruising	[] []	Depression	[] []
Hearing loss	[] []	Diarrhea	[] []	Lymph: swelling	[] []	Hallucinations	[] []
Tinnitus	[] []	Heartburn	[] []	Endo: polyuria	[] []	All/Imm: hayfever	[] []
						Runny nose	[] []

Other ROS: _____

Past Medical History:
_____
_____
_____
_____
_____
_____
_____

Past Surgical History:
_____
_____
_____
_____

Family History:
_____
_____

[] All other ROS reviewed and were NEGATIVE

Social History:
_____

Cigs: [] No Yes [] → Pack yrs _____
ETOH [] No Yes [] → Amount? _____
Illicits [] No Yes [] → Type? _____
Allergies: [] NKDA _____
Medications:
_____
_____
_____
_____
_____
_____
_____
_____
_____

Physical Exam T _____ BP _____ HR _____ Wt _____(lbs) Ht _____(in) BMI _____

Eyes	[] nl conjunctiva & lids	**ENT** External	[] no scars, lesions, masses	**Neck** External	[] no tracheal deviation
Pupils	[] equal, round, & reactive	Otoscopic	[] nl canals, TM	Palpation	[] no masses
Fundus	[] nl discs and vessels	Hearing	[] nl hearing	Thyroid	[] no enlargement
Vision	[] acuity & gross fields intact	Oropharynx	[] nl teeth, tongue, pharynx	Abnormals:	
Abnormals:		Abnormals:			

GI Palpation	[] no masses or tenderness [] no hep/splenomegaly	**Resp** Effort	[] nl w/o retractions	**Skin**	[] no rashes, or lesions
		Percussion	[] no dullness	Chest	[] nl breast, no d/c
Ausculation	[] nl bowel sounds	Palpation	[] no fremitus	Lymph nodes	[] no axillary, inguinal, cervical or submandibular LAD
Percussion	[] no dullness	Ausculation	[] CTA w/o W, R, or R		
Anus/rectum	[] no abnormality or masses [] heme negative stool	Abnormals:		GU	[] nl male/female exam
Abnormals:				Psych	[] nl cognition

CV Palpation	[] PMI nondisplaced	**Neuro** Orientation	[] AAO x 3	Abnormals:	
Auscultation	[] no murmur, gallop, or rub	Cranial nerves	[] CN II-XII intact		
Carotids	[] nl intensity w/o bruit	Sensory	[] nl sensation		
JVD	[] no jugulovenous distention	Reflexes	[] 2+ & symmetrical		
Pulses	[] 2+/= femoral & pedal pulses	Abnormals:			
Edema	[] no pedal edema				
Abnormals					

Musculoskeletal Inspection ROM Strength Tone (✓ if normal) Abnormals: **Other:**

	Inspection	ROM	Strength	Tone
Upper extremity	[]	[]	[]	[]
Lower extremity	[]	[]	[]	[]

Gait   [] nl gait and FROM

Labs:

Assessment & Plan:
_____
_____
_____
_____
_____
_____
_____
_____
_____
_____
_____
_____

Clinical Rotation_____ Date: _____

Chief Complaint:
_____

History of Present Illness:
_____
_____
_____
_____
_____

Review of Systems:

	Yes	No		Yes	No		Yes	No		Yes	No
General: fatigue	[]	[]	CV: chest pain	[]	[]	Bloody stool	[]	[]	Polydypsia	[]	[]
Weight loss	[]	[]	Edema	[]	[]	GU: dysuria	[]	[]	Polyphagia	[]	[]
Fever	[]	[]	PND	[]	[]	Frequency	[]	[]	Polyphagia	[]	[]
Chills	[]	[]	Orthopnea	[]	[]	Hematuria	[]	[]	Temp int	[]	[]
Night sweats	[]	[]	Palpitations	[]	[]	Discharge	[]	[]	Derm: rash	[]	[]
Eye: vision change	[]	[]	Claudication	[]	[]	Flank pain	[]	[]	Pruritis	[]	[]
Pain	[]	[]	Resp: cough	[]	[]	MS: arthralgia	[]	[]	Neuro: weakness	[]	[]
Redness	[]	[]	SOB	[]	[]	Arthritis	[]	[]	Seizures	[]	[]
ENT: headaches	[]	[]	Wheezing	[]	[]	Joint swelling	[]	[]	Parasthesias	[]	[]
Hoarseness	[]	[]	Hemoptysis	[]	[]	Myalgias	[]	[]	Tremors	[]	[]
Sore throat	[]	[]	GI: abd pain	[]	[]	Back pain	[]	[]	Syncope	[]	[]
Epistaxis	[]	[]	BM changes	[]	[]	Heme: bleeding	[]	[]	Psych: anxiety	[]	[]
Sinus Sx	[]	[]	N/V	[]	[]	Bruising	[]	[]	Depression	[]	[]
Hearing loss	[]	[]	Diarrhea	[]	[]	Lymph: swelling	[]	[]	Hallucinations	[]	[]
Tinnitus	[]	[]	Heartburn	[]	[]	Endo: polyuria	[]	[]	All/Imm: hayfever	[]	[]
									Runny nose	[]	[]

Other ROS: _____

Past Medical History:
_____
_____
_____
_____
_____
_____

Past Surgical History:
_____
_____
_____
_____

Family History:
_____
_____

[] All other ROS reviewed and were NEGATIVE

Social History:
_____

Cigs: [] No Yes [] → Pack yrs _____
ETOH [] No Yes [] → Amount? _____
Illicits [] No Yes [] → Type? _____
Allergies: [] NKDA _____
Medications:
_____
_____
_____
_____
_____
_____
_____
_____
_____
_____

Physical Exam T _____ BP _____ HR _____ Wt _____ (lbs) Ht _____ (in) BMI _____		
Eyes [] nl conjunctiva & lids	**ENT** External [] no scars, lesions, masses	**Neck** External [] no tracheal deviation
Pupils [] equal, round, & reactive	Otoscopic [] nl canals, TM	Palpation [] no masses
Fundus [] nl discs and vessels	Hearing [] nl hearing	Thyroid [] no enlargement
Vision [] acuity & gross fields intact	Oropharynx [] nl teeth, tongue, pharynx	Abnormals:
Abnormals:	Abnormals:	
GI Palpation [] no masses or tenderness [] no hep/splenomegaly	**Resp** Effort [] nl w/o retractions	**Skin** [] no rashes, or lesions
Ausculation [] nl bowel sounds	Percussion [] no dullness	Chest [] nl breast, no d/c
Percussion [] no dullness	Palpation [] no fremitus	Lymph nodes [] no axillary, inguinal, cervical or submandibular LAD
Anus/rectum [] no abnormality or masses [] heme negative stool	Ausculation [] CTA w/o W, R, or R	GU [] nl male/female exam
Abnormals:	Abnormals:	Psych [] nl cognition
CV Palpation [] PMI nondisplaced	**Neuro** Orientation [] AAO x 3	Abnormals:
Auscultation [] no murmur, gallop, or rub	Cranial nerves [] CN II-XII intact	
Carotids [] nl intensity w/o bruit	Sensory [] nl sensation	
JVD [] no jugulovenous distention	Reflexes [] 2+ & symmetrical	
Pulses [] 2+/= femoral & pedal pulses	Abnormals:	
Edema [] no pedal edema		
Abnormals		

Musculoskeletal Inspection ROM Strength Tone (✓ if normal) Abnormals:		**Other:**
Upper extremity [] [] [] [] Lower extremity [] [] [] []		
Gait [] nl gait and FROM		

Labs:

Assessment & Plan:

_____
_____
_____
_____
_____
_____
_____
_____
_____
_____
_____

Clinical Rotation_____   Date: _____

Chief Complaint:

_____

History of Present Illness:

_____
_____
_____
_____
_____

Review of Systems:

	Yes	No		Yes	No		Yes	No		Yes	No
General: fatigue	[]	[]	CV: chest pain	[]	[]	Bloody stool	[]	[]	Polydypsia	[]	[]
Weight loss	[]	[]	Edema	[]	[]	GU: dysuria	[]	[]	Polyphagia	[]	[]
Fever	[]	[]	PND	[]	[]	Frequency	[]	[]	Polyphagia	[]	[]
Chills	[]	[]	Orthopnea	[]	[]	Hematuria	[]	[]	Temp int	[]	[]
Night sweats	[]	[]	Palpitations	[]	[]	Discharge	[]	[]	Derm: rash	[]	[]
Eye: vision change	[]	[]	Claudication	[]	[]	Flank pain	[]	[]	Pruritis	[]	[]
Pain	[]	[]	Resp: cough	[]	[]	MS: arthralgia	[]	[]	Neuro: weakness	[]	[]
Redness	[]	[]	SOB	[]	[]	Arthritis	[]	[]	Seizures	[]	[]
ENT: headaches	[]	[]	Wheezing	[]	[]	Joint swelling	[]	[]	Parasthesias	[]	[]
Hoarseness	[]	[]	Hemoptysis	[]	[]	Myalgias	[]	[]	Tremors	[]	[]
Sore throat	[]	[]	GI: abd pain	[]	[]	Back pain	[]	[]	Syncope	[]	[]
Epistaxis	[]	[]	BM changes	[]	[]	Heme: bleeding	[]	[]	Psych: anxiety	[]	[]
Sinus Sx	[]	[]	N/V	[]	[]	Bruising	[]	[]	Depression	[]	[]
Hearing loss	[]	[]	Diarrhea	[]	[]	Lymph: swelling	[]	[]	Hallucinations	[]	[]
Tinnitus	[]	[]	Heartburn	[]	[]	Endo: polyuria	[]	[]	All/Imm: hayfever	[]	[]
									Runny nose	[]	[]

Other ROS: _____

Past Medical History:

Social History:

_____

Cigs: [] No Yes [] → Pack yrs _____
ETOH [] No Yes [] → Amount? _____
Illicits [] No Yes [] → Type? _____
Allergies: [] NKDA _____
Medications:

Past Medical History lines:
_____
_____
_____
_____
_____
_____

Past Surgical History:

_____
_____
_____
_____

Family History:

_____
_____
_____

[] All other ROS reviewed and were NEGATIVE

Physical Exam T _____ BP _____ HR _____ Wt _____(lbs) Ht _____(in) BMI _____		

Physical Exam T _____ BP _____ HR _____ Wt _____(lbs) Ht _____(in) BMI _____

Eyes	[] nl conjunctiva & lids	ENT External	[] no scars, lesions, masses	Neck External	[] no tracheal deviation
Pupils	[] equal, round, & reactive	Otoscopic	[] nl canals, TM	Palpation	[] no masses
Fundus	[] nl discs and vessels	Hearing	[] nl hearing	Thyroid	[] no enlargement
Vision	[] acuity & gross fields intact	Oropharynx	[] nl teeth, tongue, pharynx	Abnormals:	
Abnormals:		Abnormals:			

GI Palpation	[] no masses or tenderness [] no hep/splenomegaly	Resp Effort	[] nl w/o retractions	Skin	[] no rashes, or lesions
		Percussion	[] no dullness	Chest	[] nl breast, no d/c
Ausculation	[] nl bowel sounds	Palpation	[] no fremitus	Lymph nodes	[] no axillary, inguinal, cervical or submandibular LAD
Percussion	[] no dullness	Ausculation	[] CTA w/o W, R, or R		
Anus/rectum	[] no abnormality or masses [] heme negative stool	Abnormals:		GU	[] nl male/female exam
Abnormals:				Psych	[] nl cognition

CV Palpation	[] PMI nondisplaced	Neuro Orientation	[] AAO x 3	Abnormals:	
Auscultation	[] no murmur, gallop, or rub	Cranial nerves	[] CN II-XII intact		
Carotids	[] nl intensity w/o bruit	Sensory	[] nl sensation		
JVD	[] no jugulovenous distention	Reflexes	[] 2+ & symmetrical		
Pulses	[] 2+/= femoral & pedal pulses	Abnormals:			
Edema	[] no pedal edema				
Abnormals					

Musculoskeletal	Inspection	ROM	Strength	Tone (✓ if normal)	Abnormals:	Other:
Upper extremity	[]	[]	[]	[]		
Lower extremity	[]	[]	[]	[]		
Gait	[] nl gait and FROM					

Labs:

Assessment & Plan:

_____
_____
_____
_____
_____
_____
_____
_____
_____
_____
_____
_____

Clinical Rotation_____   Date: _____

Chief Complaint:
_____

History of Present Illness:
_____
_____
_____
_____
_____
_____

Review of Systems:

	Yes	No		Yes	No		Yes	No		Yes	No
General: fatigue	[]	[]	CV: chest pain	[]	[]	Bloody stool	[]	[]	Polydypsia	[]	[]
Weight loss	[]	[]	Edema	[]	[]	GU: dysuria	[]	[]	Polyphagia	[]	[]
Fever	[]	[]	PND	[]	[]	Frequency	[]	[]	Polyphagia	[]	[]
Chills	[]	[]	Orthopnea	[]	[]	Hematuria	[]	[]	Temp int	[]	[]
Night sweats	[]	[]	Palpitations	[]	[]	Discharge	[]	[]	Derm: rash	[]	[]
Eye: vision change	[]	[]	Claudication	[]	[]	Flank pain	[]	[]	Pruritis	[]	[]
Pain	[]	[]	Resp: cough	[]	[]	MS: arthralgia	[]	[]	Neuro: weakness	[]	[]
Redness	[]	[]	SOB	[]	[]	Arthritis	[]	[]	Seizures	[]	[]
ENT: headaches	[]	[]	Wheezing	[]	[]	Joint swelling	[]	[]	Parasthesias	[]	[]
Hoarseness	[]	[]	Hemoptysis	[]	[]	Myalgias	[]	[]	Tremors	[]	[]
Sore throat	[]	[]	GI: abd pain	[]	[]	Back pain	[]	[]	Syncope	[]	[]
Epistaxis	[]	[]	BM changes	[]	[]	Heme: bleeding	[]	[]	Psych: anxiety	[]	[]
Sinus Sx	[]	[]	N/V	[]	[]	Bruising	[]	[]	Depression	[]	[]
Hearing loss	[]	[]	Diarrhea	[]	[]	Lymph: swelling	[]	[]	Hallucinations	[]	[]
Tinnitus	[]	[]	Heartburn	[]	[]	Endo: polyuria	[]	[]	All/Imm: hayfever	[]	[]
									Runny nose	[]	[]

Other ROS: _____

Past Medical History:
_____
_____
_____
_____
_____
_____
_____

Social History:
_____

Cigs: [] No Yes [] → Pack yrs _____
ETOH [] No Yes [] → Amount? _____
Illicits [] No Yes [] → Type? _____
Allergies: [] NKDA _____
Medications:
_____

Past Surgical History:
_____
_____
_____
_____

Family History:
_____
_____
_____

[] All other ROS reviewed and were NEGATIVE

Physical Exam	T _____	BP _____	HR _____	Wt _____(lbs)	Ht _____(in)	BMI _____

Eyes			**ENT** External		**Neck** External	

Eyes
[] nl conjunctiva & lids

Pupils   [] equal, round, & reactive

Fundus   [] nl discs and vessels

Vision   [] acuity & gross fields intact

Abnormals:

ENT External   [] no scars, lesions, masses

Otoscopic   [] nl canals, TM

Hearing   [] nl hearing

Oropharynx   [] nl teeth, tongue, pharynx

Abnormals:

Neck External   [] no tracheal deviation

Palpation   [] no masses

Thyroid   [] no enlargement

Abnormals:

GI Palpation [] no masses or tenderness
      [] no hep/splenomegaly

Ausculation   [] nl bowel sounds

Percussion   [] no dullness

Anus/rectum   [] no abnormality or masses
      [] heme negative stool

Abnormals:

Resp Effort   [] nl w/o retractions

Percussion   [] no dullness

Palpation   [] no fremitus

Ausculation   [] CTA w/o W, R, or R

Abnormals:

Skin   [] no rashes, or lesions

Chest   [] nl breast, no d/c

Lymph nodes   [] no axillary, inguinal, cervical or submandibular LAD

GU   [] nl male/female exam

Psych   [] nl cognition

Abnormals:

CV Palpation [] PMI nondisplaced

Auscultation   [] no murmur, gallop, or rub

Carotids   [] nl intensity w/o bruit

JVD   [] no jugulovenous distention

Pulses   [] 2+/= femoral & pedal pulses

Edema   [] no pedal edema

Abnormals

Neuro   Orientation [] AAO x 3

Cranial nerves   [] CN II-XII intact

Sensory   [] nl sensation

Reflexes   [] 2+ & symmetrical

Abnormals:

Musculoskeletal   Inspection   ROM   Strength   Tone   (✓ if normal)   Abnormals:

	Inspection	ROM	Strength	Tone
Upper extremity	[]	[]	[]	[]
Lower extremity	[]	[]	[]	[]

Gait   [] nl gait and FROM

Other:

Labs:

Assessment & Plan:
_____
_____
_____
_____
_____
_____
_____
_____
_____
_____
_____

Clinical Rotation_____   Date: _____

Chief Complaint:
_____

History of Present Illness:
_____
_____
_____
_____
_____

Review of Systems:

	Yes	No		Yes	No		Yes	No		Yes	No
General: fatigue	[]	[]	CV: chest pain	[]	[]	Bloody stool	[]	[]	Polydypsia	[]	[]
Weight loss	[]	[]	Edema	[]	[]	GU: dysuria	[]	[]	Polyphagia	[]	[]
Fever	[]	[]	PND	[]	[]	Frequency	[]	[]	Polyphagia	[]	[]
Chills	[]	[]	Orthopnea	[]	[]	Hematuria	[]	[]	Temp int	[]	[]
Night sweats	[]	[]	Palpitations	[]	[]	Discharge	[]	[]	Derm: rash	[]	[]
Eye: vision change	[]	[]	Claudication	[]	[]	Flank pain	[]	[]	Pruritis	[]	[]
Pain	[]	[]	Resp: cough	[]	[]	MS: arthralgia	[]	[]	Neuro: weakness	[]	[]
Redness	[]	[]	SOB	[]	[]	Arthritis	[]	[]	Seizures	[]	[]
ENT: headaches	[]	[]	Wheezing	[]	[]	Joint swelling	[]	[]	Parasthesias	[]	[]
Hoarseness	[]	[]	Hemoptysis	[]	[]	Myalgias	[]	[]	Tremors	[]	[]
Sore throat	[]	[]	GI: abd pain	[]	[]	Back pain	[]	[]	Syncope	[]	[]
Epistaxis	[]	[]	BM changes	[]	[]	Heme: bleeding	[]	[]	Psych: anxiety	[]	[]
Sinus Sx	[]	[]	N/V	[]	[]	Bruising	[]	[]	Depression	[]	[]
Hearing loss	[]	[]	Diarrhea	[]	[]	Lymph: swelling	[]	[]	Hallucinations	[]	[]
Tinnitus	[]	[]	Heartburn	[]	[]	Endo: polyuria	[]	[]	All/Imm: hayfever	[]	[]
									Runny nose	[]	[]

Other ROS: _____

Past Medical History:
_____
_____
_____
_____
_____
_____

Past Surgical History:
_____
_____
_____
_____

Family History:
_____
_____

[] All other ROS reviewed and were NEGATIVE

Social History:
_____

Cigs: [] No Yes [] → Pack yrs _____
ETOH [] No Yes [] → Amount? _____
Illicits [] No Yes [] → Type?   _____
Allergies: [] NKDA _____
Medications:
_____
_____
_____
_____
_____
_____
_____
_____
_____
_____

Physical Exam	T _____	BP _____	HR _____	Wt _____(lbs)	Ht _____(in)	BMI _____

Eyes	[] nl conjunctiva & lids	**ENT** External	[] no scars, lesions, masses	**Neck** External	[] no tracheal deviation
Pupils	[] equal, round, & reactive	Otoscopic	[] nl canals, TM	Palpation	[] no masses
Fundus	[] nl discs and vessels	Hearing	[] nl hearing	Thyroid	[] no enlargement
Vision	[] acuity & gross fields intact	Oropharynx	[] nl teeth, tongue, pharynx	Abnormals:	
Abnormals:		Abnormals:			

GI Palpation	[] no masses or tenderness [] no hep/splenomegaly	**Resp** Effort	[] nl w/o retractions	**Skin**	[] no rashes, or lesions
Ausculation	[] nl bowel sounds	Percussion	[] no dullness	Chest	[] nl breast, no d/c
Percussion	[] no dullness	Palpation	[] no fremitus	Lymph nodes	[] no axillary, inguinal, cervical or submandibular LAD
Anus/rectum	[] no abnormality or masses [] heme negative stool	Ausculation	[] CTA w/o W, R, or R	GU	[] nl male/female exam
Abnormals:		Abnormals:		Psych	[] nl cognition

CV Palpation	[] PMI nondisplaced	**Neuro** Orientation	[] AAO x 3	Abnormals:	
Auscultation	[] no murmur, gallop, or rub	Cranial nerves	[] CN II-XII intact		
Carotids	[] nl intensity w/o bruit	Sensory	[] nl sensation		
JVD	[] no juglovenous distention	Reflexes	[] 2+ & symmetrical		
Pulses	[] 2+/= femoral & pedal pulses	Abnormals:			
Edema	[] no pedal edema				
Abnormals					

Musculoskeletal	Inspection	ROM	Strength	Tone (✓ if normal)	Abnormals:	**Other:**
Upper extremity	[]	[]	[]	[]		
Lower extremity	[]	[]	[]	[]		
Gait	[] nl gait and FROM					

Labs:

Assessment & Plan:

Clinical Rotation_____   Date: _____

Chief Complaint:

_____

History of Present Illness:

_____
_____
_____
_____
_____

Review of Systems:

	Yes	No		Yes	No		Yes	No		Yes	No
General: fatigue	[]	[]	CV: chest pain	[]	[]	Bloody stool	[]	[]	Polydypsia	[]	[]
Weight loss	[]	[]	Edema	[]	[]	GU: dysuria	[]	[]	Polyphagia	[]	[]
Fever	[]	[]	PND	[]	[]	Frequency	[]	[]	Polyphagia	[]	[]
Chills	[]	[]	Orthopnea	[]	[]	Hematuria	[]	[]	Temp int	[]	[]
Night sweats	[]	[]	Palpitations	[]	[]	Discharge	[]	[]	Derm: rash	[]	[]
Eye: vision change	[]	[]	Claudication	[]	[]	Flank pain	[]	[]	Pruritis	[]	[]
Pain	[]	[]	Resp: cough	[]	[]	MS: arthralgia	[]	[]	Neuro: weakness	[]	[]
Redness	[]	[]	SOB	[]	[]	Arthritis	[]	[]	Seizures	[]	[]
ENT: headaches	[]	[]	Wheezing	[]	[]	Joint swelling	[]	[]	Parasthesias	[]	[]
Hoarseness	[]	[]	Hemoptysis	[]	[]	Myalgias	[]	[]	Tremors	[]	[]
Sore throat	[]	[]	GI: abd pain	[]	[]	Back pain	[]	[]	Syncope	[]	[]
Epistaxis	[]	[]	BM changes	[]	[]	Heme: bleeding	[]	[]	Psych: anxiety	[]	[]
Sinus Sx	[]	[]	N/V	[]	[]	Bruising	[]	[]	Depression	[]	[]
Hearing loss	[]	[]	Diarrhea	[]	[]	Lymph: swelling	[]	[]	Hallucinations	[]	[]
Tinnitus	[]	[]	Heartburn	[]	[]	Endo: polyuria	[]	[]	All/Imm: hayfever	[]	[]
									Runny nose	[]	[]

Other ROS: _____

Past Medical History:

_____
_____
_____
_____
_____
_____

Past Surgical History:

_____
_____
_____
_____

Family History:

_____

[] All other ROS reviewed and were NEGATIVE

Social History:

_____

Cigs: [] No Yes [] → Pack yrs _____
ETOH [] No Yes [] → Amount? _____
Illicits [] No Yes [] → Type? _____
Allergies: [] NKDA _____
Medications:

_____
_____
_____
_____
_____
_____
_____
_____

| **Physical Exam** T _____ | BP _____ | HR _____ | Wt _____(lbs) | Ht _____(in) BMI _____ |

Eyes [] nl conjunctiva & lids	**ENT** External [] no scars, lesions, masses	**Neck** External [] no tracheal deviation
Pupils [] equal, round, & reactive	Otoscopic [] nl canals, TM	Palpation [] no masses
Fundus [] nl discs and vessels	Hearing [] nl hearing	Thyroid [] no enlargement
Vision [] acuity & gross fields intact	Oropharynx [] nl teeth, tongue, pharynx	Abnormals:
Abnormals:	Abnormals:	
GI Palpation [] no masses or tenderness [] no hep/splenomegaly	**Resp** Effort [] nl w/o retractions	**Skin** [] no rashes, or lesions
	Percussion [] no dullness	Chest [] nl breast, no d/c
Ausculation [] nl bowel sounds	Palpation [] no fremitus	Lymph nodes [] no axillary, inguinal, cervical or submandibular LAD
Percussion [] no dullness	Ausculation [] CTA w/o W, R, or R	
Anus/rectum [] no abnormality or masses [] heme negative stool	Abnormals:	GU [] nl male/female exam
Abnormals:		Psych [] nl cognition
CV Palpation [] PMI nondisplaced	**Neuro** Orientation [] AAO x 3	Abnormals:
Auscultation [] no murmur, gallop, or rub	Cranial nerves [] CN II-XII intact	
Carotids [] nl intensity w/o bruit	Sensory [] nl sensation	
JVD [] no jugulovenous distention	Reflexes [] 2+ & symmetrical	
Pulses [] 2+/= femoral & pedal pulses	Abnormals:	
Edema [] no pedal edema		
Abnormals		

Musculoskeletal Inspection ROM Strength Tone (✓ if normal) Abnormals:	**Other:**
Upper extremity [] [] [] [] Lower extremity [] [] [] []	
Gait [] nl gait and FROM	

Labs:

Assessment & Plan:

_____
_____
_____
_____
_____
_____
_____
_____
_____
_____
_____
_____

Clinical Rotation_____   Date: _____

Chief Complaint:

_____

History of Present Illness:

_____
_____
_____
_____
_____

Review of Systems:

	Yes	No		Yes	No		Yes	No		Yes	No
General: fatigue	[]	[]	CV: chest pain	[]	[]	Bloody stool	[]	[]	Polydypsia	[]	[]
Weight loss	[]	[]	Edema	[]	[]	GU: dysuria	[]	[]	Polyphagia	[]	[]
Fever	[]	[]	PND	[]	[]	Frequency	[]	[]	Polyphagia	[]	[]
Chills	[]	[]	Orthopnea	[]	[]	Hematuria	[]	[]	Temp int	[]	[]
Night sweats	[]	[]	Palpitations	[]	[]	Discharge	[]	[]	Derm: rash	[]	[]
Eye: vision change	[]	[]	Claudication	[]	[]	Flank pain	[]	[]	Pruritis	[]	[]
Pain	[]	[]	Resp: cough	[]	[]	MS: arthralgia	[]	[]	Neuro: weakness	[]	[]
Redness	[]	[]	SOB	[]	[]	Arthritis	[]	[]	Seizures	[]	[]
ENT: headaches	[]	[]	Wheezing	[]	[]	Joint swelling	[]	[]	Parasthesias	[]	[]
Hoarseness	[]	[]	Hemoptysis	[]	[]	Myalgias	[]	[]	Tremors	[]	[]
Sore throat	[]	[]	GI: abd pain	[]	[]	Back pain	[]	[]	Syncope	[]	[]
Epistaxis	[]	[]	BM changes	[]	[]	Heme: bleeding	[]	[]	Psych: anxiety	[]	[]
Sinus Sx	[]	[]	N/V	[]	[]	Bruising	[]	[]	Depression	[]	[]
Hearing loss	[]	[]	Diarrhea	[]	[]	Lymph: swelling	[]	[]	Hallucinations	[]	[]
Tinnitus	[]	[]	Heartburn	[]	[]	Endo: polyuria	[]	[]	All/Imm: hayfever	[]	[]
									Runny nose	[]	[]

Other ROS: _____

Past Medical History:

_____
_____
_____
_____
_____
_____

Past Surgical History:

_____
_____
_____

Family History:

_____
_____

[ ] All other ROS reviewed and were NEGATIVE

Social History:

_____

Cigs: [] No Yes [] → Pack yrs _____
ETOH [] No Yes [] → Amount? _____
Illicits [] No Yes [] → Type? _____
Allergies: [] NKDA _____
Medications:

_____
_____
_____
_____
_____
_____
_____
_____
_____

Physical Exam   T _____   BP _____   HR _____   Wt _____ (lbs)   Ht _____ (in)   BMI _____

Eyes	[] nl conjunctiva & lids	**ENT** External	[] no scars, lesions, masses	**Neck** External	[] no tracheal deviation
Pupils	[] equal, round, & reactive	Otoscopic	[] nl canals, TM	Palpation	[] no masses
Fundus	[] nl discs and vessels	Hearing	[] nl hearing	Thyroid	[] no enlargement
Vision	[] acuity & gross fields intact	Oropharynx	[] nl teeth, tongue, pharynx	Abnormals:	
Abnormals:		Abnormals:			

GI Palpation	[] no masses or tenderness [] no hep/splenomegaly	**Resp** Effort	[] nl w/o retractions	**Skin**	[] no rashes, or lesions
Ausculation	[] nl bowel sounds	Percussion	[] no dullness	Chest	[] nl breast, no d/c
Percussion	[] no dullness	Palpation	[] no fremitus	Lymph nodes	[] no axillary, inguinal, cervical or submandibular LAD
Anus/rectum	[] no abnormality or masses [] heme negative stool	Ausculation	[] CTA w/o W, R, or R	GU	[] nl male/female exam
Abnormals:		Abnormals:		Psych	[] nl cognition

CV Palpation	[] PMI nondisplaced	**Neuro** Orientation	[] AAO x 3	Abnormals:	
Auscultation	[] no murmur, gallop, or rub	Cranial nerves	[] CN II-XII intact		
Carotids	[] nl intensity w/o bruit	Sensory	[] nl sensation		
JVD	[] no jugulovenous distention	Reflexes	[] 2+ & symmetrical		
Pulses	[] 2+/= femoral & pedal pulses	Abnormals:			
Edema	[] no pedal edema				
Abnormals					

Musculoskeletal	Inspection	ROM	Strength	Tone (✓ if normal)	Abnormals:	**Other:**
Upper extremity	[]	[]	[]	[]		
Lower extremity	[]	[]	[]	[]		
Gait	[] nl gait and FROM					

Labs:

Assessment & Plan:

_____
_____
_____
_____
_____
_____
_____
_____
_____
_____
_____

Clinical Rotation_____

Date: _____

Chief Complaint:

_____

History of Present Illness:

_____
_____
_____
_____
_____

Review of Systems:

	Yes	No		Yes	No		Yes	No		Yes	No
General: fatigue	[]	[]	CV: chest pain	[]	[]	Bloody stool	[]	[]	Polydypsia	[]	[]
Weight loss	[]	[]	Edema	[]	[]	GU: dysuria	[]	[]	Polyphagia	[]	[]
Fever	[]	[]	PND	[]	[]	Frequency	[]	[]	Polyphagia	[]	[]
Chills	[]	[]	Orthopnea	[]	[]	Hematuria	[]	[]	Temp int	[]	[]
Night sweats	[]	[]	Palpitations	[]	[]	Discharge	[]	[]	Derm: rash	[]	[]
Eye: vision change	[]	[]	Claudication	[]	[]	Flank pain	[]	[]	Pruritis	[]	[]
Pain	[]	[]	Resp: cough	[]	[]	MS: arthralgia	[]	[]	Neuro: weakness	[]	[]
Redness	[]	[]	SOB	[]	[]	Arthritis	[]	[]	Seizures	[]	[]
ENT: headaches	[]	[]	Wheezing	[]	[]	Joint swelling	[]	[]	Parasthesias	[]	[]
Hoarseness	[]	[]	Hemoptysis	[]	[]	Myalgias	[]	[]	Tremors	[]	[]
Sore throat	[]	[]	GI: abd pain	[]	[]	Back pain	[]	[]	Syncope	[]	[]
Epistaxis	[]	[]	BM changes	[]	[]	Heme: bleeding	[]	[]	Psych: anxiety	[]	[]
Sinus Sx	[]	[]	N/V	[]	[]	Bruising	[]	[]	Depression	[]	[]
Hearing loss	[]	[]	Diarrhea	[]	[]	Lymph: swelling	[]	[]	Hallucinations	[]	[]
Tinnitus	[]	[]	Heartburn	[]	[]	Endo: polyuria	[]	[]	All/Imm: hayfever	[]	[]
									Runny nose	[]	[]

Other ROS: _____

Past Medical History:

_____
_____
_____
_____
_____
_____

Past Surgical History:

_____
_____
_____
_____

Family History:

_____
_____

[] All other ROS reviewed and were NEGATIVE

Social History:

_____

Cigs: [] No Yes [] → Pack yrs _____
ETOH [] No Yes [] → Amount? _____
Illicits [] No Yes [] → Type? _____
Allergies: [] NKDA _____
Medications:

_____
_____
_____
_____
_____
_____
_____
_____
_____

Physical Exam T _____ BP _____ HR _____ Wt _____(lbs) Ht _____(in) BMI _____

Eyes	[] nl conjunctiva & lids	ENT External	[] no scars, lesions, masses	Neck External	[] no tracheal deviation
Pupils	[] equal, round, & reactive	Otoscopic	[] nl canals, TM	Palpation	[] no masses
Fundus	[] nl discs and vessels	Hearing	[] nl hearing	Thyroid	[] no enlargement
Vision	[] acuity & gross fields intact	Oropharynx	[] nl teeth, tongue, pharynx	Abnormals:	
Abnormals:		Abnormals:			

GI Palpation	[] no masses or tenderness [] no hep/splenomegaly	Resp Effort	[] nl w/o retractions	Skin	[] no rashes, or lesions
		Percussion	[] no dullness	Chest	[] nl breast, no d/c
Ausculation	[] nl bowel sounds	Palpation	[] no fremitus	Lymph nodes	[] no axillary, inguinal, cervical or submandibular LAD
Percussion	[] no dullness	Ausculation	[] CTA w/o W, R, or R		
Anus/rectum	[] no abnormality or masses [] heme negative stool	Abnormals:		GU	[] nl male/female exam
Abnormals:				Psych	[] nl cognition
CV Palpation	[] PMI nondisplaced	Neuro Orientation	[] AAO x 3	Abnormals:	
Auscultation	[] no murmur, gallop, or rub	Cranial nerves	[] CN II-XII intact		
Carotids	[] nl intensity w/o bruit	Sensory	[] nl sensation		
JVD	[] no jugulovenous distention	Reflexes	[] 2+ & symmetrical		
Pulses	[] 2+/= femoral & pedal pulses	Abnormals:			
Edema	[] no pedal edema				
Abnormals					

Musculoskeletal	Inspection	ROM	Strength	Tone (✓ if normal)	Abnormals:	Other:
Upper extremity	[]	[]	[]	[]		
Lower extremity	[]	[]	[]	[]		
Gait	[] nl gait and FROM					

Labs:

Assessment & Plan:

_____
_____
_____
_____
_____
_____
_____
_____
_____
_____

Clinical Rotation_____ Date: _____

Chief Complaint:

_____

History of Present Illness:

_____
_____
_____
_____
_____

Review of Systems:

	Yes	No		Yes	No		Yes	No		Yes	No
General: fatigue	[]	[]	CV: chest pain	[]	[]	Bloody stool	[]	[]	Polydypsia	[]	[]
Weight loss	[]	[]	Edema	[]	[]	GU: dysuria	[]	[]	Polyphagia	[]	[]
Fever	[]	[]	PND	[]	[]	Frequency	[]	[]	Polyphagia	[]	[]
Chills	[]	[]	Orthopnea	[]	[]	Hematuria	[]	[]	Temp int	[]	[]
Night sweats	[]	[]	Palpitations	[]	[]	Discharge	[]	[]	Derm: rash	[]	[]
Eye: vision change	[]	[]	Claudication	[]	[]	Flank pain	[]	[]	Pruritis	[]	[]
Pain	[]	[]	Resp: cough	[]	[]	MS: arthralgia	[]	[]	Neuro: weakness	[]	[]
Redness	[]	[]	SOB	[]	[]	Arthritis	[]	[]	Seizures	[]	[]
ENT: headaches	[]	[]	Wheezing	[]	[]	Joint swelling	[]	[]	Parasthesias	[]	[]
Hoarseness	[]	[]	Hemoptysis	[]	[]	Myalgias	[]	[]	Tremors	[]	[]
Sore throat	[]	[]	GI: abd pain	[]	[]	Back pain	[]	[]	Syncope	[]	[]
Epistaxis	[]	[]	BM changes	[]	[]	Heme: bleeding	[]	[]	Psych: anxiety	[]	[]
Sinus Sx	[]	[]	N/V	[]	[]	Bruising	[]	[]	Depression	[]	[]
Hearing loss	[]	[]	Diarrhea	[]	[]	Lymph: swelling	[]	[]	Hallucinations	[]	[]
Tinnitus	[]	[]	Heartburn	[]	[]	Endo: polyuria	[]	[]	All/Imm: hayfever	[]	[]
									Runny nose	[]	[]

Other ROS: _____

Past Medical History:

_____
_____
_____
_____
_____
_____

Past Surgical History:

_____
_____
_____

Family History:

_____
_____

[] All other ROS reviewed and were NEGATIVE

Social History:

_____

Cigs: [] No Yes [] → Pack yrs _____
ETOH [] No Yes [] → Amount? _____
Illicits [] No Yes [] → Type? _____
Allergies: [] NKDA _____
Medications:

_____
_____
_____
_____
_____
_____
_____
_____
_____

Physical Exam	T _____	BP _____	HR _____	Wt _____(lbs)	Ht _____(in)	BMI _____

Eyes [] nl conjunctiva & lids

Pupils [] equal, round, & reactive

Fundus [] nl discs and vessels

Vision [] acuity & gross fields intact

Abnormals:

ENT External [] no scars, lesions, masses

Otoscopic [] nl canals, TM

Hearing [] nl hearing

Oropharynx [] nl teeth, tongue, pharynx

Abnormals:

Neck External [] no tracheal deviation

Palpation [] no masses

Thyroid [] no enlargement

Abnormals:

GI Palpation [] no masses or tenderness
[] no hep/splenomegaly

Ausculation [] nl bowel sounds

Percussion [] no dullness

Anus/rectum [] no abnormality or masses
[] heme negative stool

Abnormals:

Resp Effort [] nl w/o retractions

Percussion [] no dullness

Palpation [] no fremitus

Ausculation [] CTA w/o W, R, or R

Abnormals:

Skin [] no rashes, or lesions

Chest [] nl breast, no d/c

Lymph nodes [] no axillary, inguinal, cervical or submandibular LAD

GU [] nl male/female exam

Psych [] nl cognition

Abnormals:

CV Palpation [] PMI nondisplaced

Auscultation [] no murmur, gallop, or rub

Carotids [] nl intensity w/o bruit

JVD [] no jugulovenous distention

Pulses [] 2+/= femoral & pedal pulses

Edema [] no pedal edema

Abnormals

Neuro Orientation [] AAO x 3

Cranial nerves [] CN II-XII intact

Sensory [] nl sensation

Reflexes [] 2+ & symmetrical

Abnormals:

Musculoskeletal Inspection ROM Strength Tone (✓ if normal) Abnormals:	**Other:**

Upper extremity [] [] [] []
Lower extremity [] [] [] []

Gait [] nl gait and FROM

Labs:

Assessment & Plan:

_____
_____
_____
_____
_____
_____
_____
_____
_____
_____
_____

Clinical Rotation_____   Date: _____

Chief Complaint:

_____

History of Present Illness:

_____
_____
_____
_____
_____

Review of Systems:

	Yes	No		Yes	No		Yes	No		Yes	No
General: fatigue	[]	[]	CV: chest pain	[]	[]	Bloody stool	[]	[]	Polydypsia	[]	[]
Weight loss	[]	[]	Edema	[]	[]	GU: dysuria	[]	[]	Polyphagia	[]	[]
Fever	[]	[]	PND	[]	[]	Frequency	[]	[]	Polyphagia	[]	[]
Chills	[]	[]	Orthopnea	[]	[]	Hematuria	[]	[]	Temp int	[]	[]
Night sweats	[]	[]	Palpitations	[]	[]	Discharge	[]	[]	Derm: rash	[]	[]
Eye: vision change	[]	[]	Claudication	[]	[]	Flank pain	[]	[]	Pruritis	[]	[]
Pain	[]	[]	Resp: cough	[]	[]	MS: arthralgia	[]	[]	Neuro: weakness	[]	[]
Redness	[]	[]	SOB	[]	[]	Arthritis	[]	[]	Seizures	[]	[]
ENT: headaches	[]	[]	Wheezing	[]	[]	Joint swelling	[]	[]	Parasthesias	[]	[]
Hoarseness	[]	[]	Hemoptysis	[]	[]	Myalgias	[]	[]	Tremors	[]	[]
Sore throat	[]	[]	GI: abd pain	[]	[]	Back pain	[]	[]	Syncope	[]	[]
Epistaxis	[]	[]	BM changes	[]	[]	Heme: bleeding	[]	[]	Psych: anxiety	[]	[]
Sinus Sx	[]	[]	N/V	[]	[]	Bruising	[]	[]	Depression	[]	[]
Hearing loss	[]	[]	Diarrhea	[]	[]	Lymph: swelling	[]	[]	Hallucinations	[]	[]
Tinnitus	[]	[]	Heartburn	[]	[]	Endo: polyuria	[]	[]	All/Imm: hayfever	[]	[]
									Runny nose	[]	[]

Other ROS: _____

Past Medical History:

_____
_____
_____
_____
_____
_____

Past Surgical History:

_____
_____
_____
_____

Family History:

_____
_____
_____

Social History:

_____

Cigs: [] No Yes [] → Pack yrs _____
ETOH [] No Yes [] → Amount? _____
Illicits [] No Yes [] → Type? _____
Allergies: [] NKDA _____
Medications:

_____
_____
_____
_____
_____
_____
_____
_____
_____
_____

[] All other ROS reviewed and were NEGATIVE

Physical Exam T _____ BP _____ HR _____ Wt _____(lbs) Ht _____(in) BMI _____

Eyes	[] nl conjunctiva & lids	**ENT** External	[] no scars, lesions, masses	**Neck** External	[] no tracheal deviation
Pupils	[] equal, round, & reactive	Otoscopic	[] nl canals, TM	Palpation	[] no masses
Fundus	[] nl discs and vessels	Hearing	[] nl hearing	Thyroid	[] no enlargement
Vision	[] acuity & gross fields intact	Oropharynx	[] nl teeth, tongue, pharynx	Abnormals:	
Abnormals:		Abnormals:			

GI Palpation [] no masses or tenderness [] no hep/splenomegaly	**Resp** Effort [] nl w/o retractions	**Skin** [] no rashes, or lesions
	Percussion [] no dullness	Chest [] nl breast, no d/c
Ausculation [] nl bowel sounds	Palpation [] no fremitus	Lymph nodes [] no axillary, inguinal, cervical or submandibular LAD
Percussion [] no dullness	Ausculation [] CTA w/o W, R, or R	
Anus/rectum [] no abnormality or masses [] heme negative stool	Abnormals:	GU [] nl male/female exam
Abnormals:		Psych [] nl cognition
CV Palpation [] PMI nondisplaced	**Neuro** Orientation [] AAO x 3	Abnormals:
Auscultation [] no murmur, gallop, or rub	Cranial nerves [] CN II-XII intact	
Carotids [] nl intensity w/o bruit	Sensory [] nl sensation	
JVD [] no jugulovenous distention	Reflexes [] 2+ & symmetrical	
Pulses [] 2+/= femoral & pedal pulses	Abnormals:	
Edema [] no pedal edema		
Abnormals		

Musculoskeletal Inspection ROM Strength Tone (✓ if normal) Abnormals:		**Other:**
Upper extremity [] [] [] []		
Lower extremity [] [] [] []		
Gait [] nl gait and FROM		

Labs:

Assessment & Plan:

_____
_____
_____
_____
_____
_____
_____
_____
_____
_____
_____

Clinical Rotation_____   Date: _____

Chief Complaint:
_____

History of Present Illness:
_____
_____
_____
_____
_____

Review of Systems:

	Yes	No		Yes	No		Yes	No		Yes	No
General: fatigue	[]	[]	CV: chest pain	[]	[]	Bloody stool	[]	[]	Polydypsia	[]	[]
Weight loss	[]	[]	Edema	[]	[]	GU: dysuria	[]	[]	Polyphagia	[]	[]
Fever	[]	[]	PND	[]	[]	Frequency	[]	[]	Polyphagia	[]	[]
Chills	[]	[]	Orthopnea	[]	[]	Hematuria	[]	[]	Temp int	[]	[]
Night sweats	[]	[]	Palpitations	[]	[]	Discharge	[]	[]	Derm: rash	[]	[]
Eye: vision change	[]	[]	Claudication	[]	[]	Flank pain	[]	[]	Pruritis	[]	[]
Pain	[]	[]	Resp: cough	[]	[]	MS: arthralgia	[]	[]	Neuro: weakness	[]	[]
Redness	[]	[]	SOB	[]	[]	Arthritis	[]	[]	Seizures	[]	[]
ENT: headaches	[]	[]	Wheezing	[]	[]	Joint swelling	[]	[]	Parasthesias	[]	[]
Hoarseness	[]	[]	Hemoptysis	[]	[]	Myalgias	[]	[]	Tremors	[]	[]
Sore throat	[]	[]	GI: abd pain	[]	[]	Back pain	[]	[]	Syncope	[]	[]
Epistaxis	[]	[]	BM changes	[]	[]	Heme: bleeding	[]	[]	Psych: anxiety	[]	[]
Sinus Sx	[]	[]	N/V	[]	[]	Bruising	[]	[]	Depression	[]	[]
Hearing loss	[]	[]	Diarrhea	[]	[]	Lymph: swelling	[]	[]	Hallucinations	[]	[]
Tinnitus	[]	[]	Heartburn	[]	[]	Endo: polyuria	[]	[]	All/Imm: hayfever	[]	[]
									Runny nose	[]	[]

Other ROS: _____

Past Medical History:
_____
_____
_____
_____
_____
_____
_____

Past Surgical History:
_____
_____
_____
_____

Family History:
_____
_____

[] All other ROS reviewed and were NEGATIVE

Social History:
_____

Cigs: [] No Yes [] → Pack yrs _____
ETOH [] No Yes [] → Amount? _____
Illicits [] No Yes [] → Type? _____
Allergies: [] NKDA _____
Medications:
_____
_____
_____
_____
_____
_____
_____
_____
_____

Physical Exam	T _____	BP _____	HR _____	Wt _____ (lbs)	Ht _____ (in)	BMI _____

Eyes			**ENT** External		**Neck** External	
Eyes	[] nl conjunctiva & lids		ENT External	[] no scars, lesions, masses	Neck External	[] no tracheal deviation
Pupils	[] equal, round, & reactive		Otoscopic	[] nl canals, TM	Palpation	[] no masses
Fundus	[] nl discs and vessels		Hearing	[] nl hearing	Thyroid	[] no enlargement
Vision	[] acuity & gross fields intact		Oropharynx	[] nl teeth, tongue, pharynx	Abnormals:	
Abnormals:			Abnormals:			

GI Palpation [] no masses or tenderness [] no hep/splenomegaly
Ausculation [] nl bowel sounds
Percussion [] no dullness
Anus/rectum [] no abnormality or masses [] heme negative stool
Abnormals:

Resp Effort [] nl w/o retractions
Percussion [] no dullness
Palpation [] no fremitus
Ausculation [] CTA w/o W, R, or R
Abnormals:

Skin [] no rashes, or lesions
Chest [] nl breast, no d/c
Lymph nodes [] no axillary, inguinal, cervical or submandibular LAD
GU [] nl male/female exam
Psych [] nl cognition
Abnormals:

CV Palpation [] PMI nondisplaced
Auscultation [] no murmur, gallop, or rub
Carotids [] nl intensity w/o bruit
JVD [] no jugulovenous distention
Pulses [] 2+/= femoral & pedal pulses
Edema [] no pedal edema
Abnormals

Neuro Orientation [] AAO x 3
Cranial nerves [] CN II-XII intact
Sensory [] nl sensation
Reflexes [] 2+ & symmetrical
Abnormals:

Musculoskeletal Inspection ROM Strength Tone (✓ if normal) Abnormals:

	Inspection	ROM	Strength	Tone
Upper extremity	[]	[]	[]	[]
Lower extremity	[]	[]	[]	[]

Gait [] nl gait and FROM

Other:

Labs:

Assessment & Plan:
_____
_____
_____
_____
_____
_____
_____
_____
_____
_____
_____

Clinical Rotation_____   Date: _____

Chief Complaint:
_____

History of Present Illness:
_____
_____
_____
_____
_____
_____

Review of Systems:

	Yes No		Yes No		Yes No		Yes No
General: fatigue	[] []	CV: chest pain	[] []	Bloody stool	[] []	Polydypsia	[] []
Weight loss	[] []	Edema	[] []	GU: dysuria	[] []	Polyphagia	[] []
Fever	[] []	PND	[] []	Frequency	[] []	Polyphagia	[] []
Chills	[] []	Orthopnea	[] []	Hematuria	[] []	Temp int	[] []
Night sweats	[] []	Palpitations	[] []	Discharge	[] []	Derm: rash	[] []
Eye: vision change	[] []	Claudication	[] []	Flank pain	[] []	Pruritis	[] []
Pain	[] []	Resp: cough	[] []	MS: arthralgia	[] []	Neuro: weakness	[] []
Redness	[] []	SOB	[] []	Arthritis	[] []	Seizures	[] []
ENT: headaches	[] []	Wheezing	[] []	Joint swelling	[] []	Parasthesias	[] []
Hoarseness	[] []	Hemoptysis	[] []	Myalgias	[] []	Tremors	[] []
Sore throat	[] []	GI: abd pain	[] []	Back pain	[] []	Syncope	[] []
Epistaxis	[] []	BM changes	[] []	Heme: bleeding	[] []	Psych: anxiety	[] []
Sinus Sx	[] []	N/V	[] []	Bruising	[] []	Depression	[] []
Hearing loss	[] []	Diarrhea	[] []	Lymph: swelling	[] []	Hallucinations	[] []
Tinnitus	[] []	Heartburn	[] []	Endo: polyuria	[] []	All/Imm: hayfever	[] []
						Runny nose	[] []

Other ROS: _____

Past Medical History:
_____
_____
_____
_____
_____
_____
_____

Past Surgical History:
_____
_____
_____
_____

Family History:
_____
_____

[] All other ROS reviewed and were NEGATIVE

Social History:
_____

Cigs: [] No Yes [] → Pack yrs _____
ETOH [] No Yes [] → Amount? _____
Illicits [] No Yes [] → Type? _____
Allergies: [] NKDA _____
Medications:
_____
_____
_____
_____
_____
_____
_____
_____
_____
_____

Physical Exam   T _____   BP _____   HR _____   Wt _____ (lbs)   Ht _____ (in)   BMI _____

Eyes	[] nl conjunctiva & lids	ENT External	[] no scars, lesions, masses	Neck External	[] no tracheal deviation
Pupils	[] equal, round, & reactive	Otoscopic	[] nl canals, TM	Palpation	[] no masses
Fundus	[] nl discs and vessels	Hearing	[] nl hearing	Thyroid	[] no enlargement
Vision	[] acuity & gross fields intact	Oropharynx	[] nl teeth, tongue, pharynx	Abnormals:	
Abnormals:		Abnormals:			

GI Palpation []	no masses or tenderness	Resp Effort	[] nl w/o retractions	Skin	[] no rashes, or lesions
[]	no hep/splenomegaly	Percussion	[] no dullness	Chest	[] nl breast, no d/c
Ausculation []	nl bowel sounds	Palpation	[] no fremitus	Lymph nodes	[] no axillary, inguinal,
Percussion []	no dullness	Ausculation	[] CTA w/o W, R, or R		cervical or submandibular LAD
Anus/rectum []	no abnormality or masses	Abnormals:		GU	[] nl male/female exam
[]	heme negative stool			Psych	[] nl cognition
Abnormals:					

CV Palpation []	PMI nondisplaced	Neuro Orientation [] AAO x 3	Abnormals:
Auscultation []	no murmur, gallop, or rub	Cranial nerves [] CN II-XII intact	
Carotids []	nl intensity w/o bruit	Sensory [] nl sensation	
JVD []	no jugulovenous distention	Reflexes [] 2+ & symmetrical	
Pulses []	2+/= femoral & pedal pulses	Abnormals:	
Edema []	no pedal edema		
Abnormals			

Musculoskeletal	Inspection	ROM	Strength	Tone	(✓ if normal)	Abnormals:	Other:
Upper extremity	[]	[]	[]	[]			
Lower extremity	[]	[]	[]	[]			
Gait	[] nl gait and FROM						

Labs:

Assessment & Plan:

_____
_____
_____
_____
_____
_____
_____
_____
_____
_____
_____

Clinical Rotation_____   Date: _____

Chief Complaint:
_____

History of Present Illness:
_____
_____
_____
_____
_____

Review of Systems:

	Yes	No		Yes	No		Yes	No		Yes	No
General: fatigue	[]	[]	CV: chest pain	[]	[]	Bloody stool	[]	[]	Polydypsia	[]	[]
Weight loss	[]	[]	Edema	[]	[]	GU: dysuria	[]	[]	Polyphagia	[]	[]
Fever	[]	[]	PND	[]	[]	Frequency	[]	[]	Polyphagia	[]	[]
Chills	[]	[]	Orthopnea	[]	[]	Hematuria	[]	[]	Temp int	[]	[]
Night sweats	[]	[]	Palpitations	[]	[]	Discharge	[]	[]	Derm: rash	[]	[]
Eye: vision change	[]	[]	Claudication	[]	[]	Flank pain	[]	[]	Pruritis	[]	[]
Pain	[]	[]	Resp: cough	[]	[]	MS: arthralgia	[]	[]	Neuro: weakness	[]	[]
Redness	[]	[]	SOB	[]	[]	Arthritis	[]	[]	Seizures	[]	[]
ENT: headaches	[]	[]	Wheezing	[]	[]	Joint swelling	[]	[]	Parasthesias	[]	[]
Hoarseness	[]	[]	Hemoptysis	[]	[]	Myalgias	[]	[]	Tremors	[]	[]
Sore throat	[]	[]	GI: abd pain	[]	[]	Back pain	[]	[]	Syncope	[]	[]
Epistaxis	[]	[]	BM changes	[]	[]	Heme: bleeding	[]	[]	Psych: anxiety	[]	[]
Sinus Sx	[]	[]	N/V	[]	[]	Bruising	[]	[]	Depression	[]	[]
Hearing loss	[]	[]	Diarrhea	[]	[]	Lymph: swelling	[]	[]	Hallucinations	[]	[]
Tinnitus	[]	[]	Heartburn	[]	[]	Endo: polyuria	[]	[]	All/Imm: hayfever	[]	[]
									Runny nose	[]	[]

Other ROS: _____

Past Medical History:
_____
_____
_____
_____
_____
_____

Past Surgical History:
_____
_____
_____
_____

Family History:
_____
_____

[] All other ROS reviewed and were NEGATIVE

Social History:
_____

Cigs: [] No Yes [] → Pack yrs _____
ETOH [] No Yes [] → Amount? _____
Illicits [] No Yes [] → Type?   _____
Allergies: [] NKDA _____
Medications:
_____
_____
_____
_____
_____
_____
_____
_____
_____
_____
_____

Physical Exam T _____ BP _____ HR _____ Wt _____(lbs) Ht _____(in) BMI _____

Eyes	[] nl conjunctiva & lids	**ENT** External	[] no scars, lesions, masses	**Neck** External	[]	no tracheal deviation
Pupils	[] equal, round, & reactive	Otoscopic	[] nl canals, TM	Palpation	[]	no masses
Fundus	[] nl discs and vessels	Hearing	[] nl hearing	Thyroid	[]	no enlargement
Vision	[] acuity & gross fields intact	Oropharynx	[] nl teeth, tongue, pharynx	Abnormals:		
Abnormals:		Abnormals:				

GI Palpation	[] no masses or tenderness [] no hep/splenomegaly	**Resp** Effort	[] nl w/o retractions	**Skin**	[]	no rashes, or lesions
Ausculation	[] nl bowel sounds	Percussion	[] no dullness	Chest	[]	nl breast, no d/c
Percussion	[] no dullness	Palpation	[] no fremitus	Lymph nodes	[]	no axillary, inguinal, cervical or submandibular LAD
Anus/rectum	[] no abnormality or masses [] heme negative stool	Ausculation	[] CTA w/o W, R, or R	GU	[]	nl male/female exam
Abnormals:		Abnormals:		Psych	[]	nl cognition

CV Palpation	[] PMI nondisplaced	**Neuro** Orientation	[] AAO x 3	Abnormals:
Auscultation	[] no murmur, gallop, or rub	Cranial nerves	[] CN II-XII intact	
Carotids	[] nl intensity w/o bruit	Sensory	[] nl sensation	
JVD	[] no jugulovenous distention	Reflexes	[] 2+ & symmetrical	
Pulses	[] 2+/= femoral & pedal pulses	Abnormals:		
Edema	[] no pedal edema			
Abnormals				

Musculoskeletal	Inspection	ROM	Strength	Tone	(✓ if normal)	Abnormals:	**Other:**
Upper extremity	[]	[]	[]	[]			
Lower extremity	[]	[]	[]	[]			
Gait	[]	nl gait and FROM					

Labs:

Assessment & Plan:

_____
_____
_____
_____
_____
_____
_____
_____
_____
_____
_____

Clinical Rotation_____   Date: _____

Chief Complaint:
_____

History of Present Illness:
_____
_____
_____
_____
_____

Review of Systems:

	Yes No		Yes No		Yes No		Yes No
General: fatigue	[] []	CV: chest pain	[] []	Bloody stool	[] []	Polydypsia	[] []
Weight loss	[] []	Edema	[] []	GU: dysuria	[] []	Polyphagia	[] []
Fever	[] []	PND	[] []	Frequency	[] []	Polyphagia	[] []
Chills	[] []	Orthopnea	[] []	Hematuria	[] []	Temp int	[] []
Night sweats	[] []	Palpitations	[] []	Discharge	[] []	Derm: rash	[] []
Eye: vision change	[] []	Claudication	[] []	Flank pain	[] []	Pruritis	[] []
Pain	[] []	Resp: cough	[] []	MS: arthralgia	[] []	Neuro: weakness	[] []
Redness	[] []	SOB	[] []	Arthritis	[] []	Seizures	[] []
ENT: headaches	[] []	Wheezing	[] []	Joint swelling	[] []	Parasthesias	[] []
Hoarseness	[] []	Hemoptysis	[] []	Myalgias	[] []	Tremors	[] []
Sore throat	[] []	GI: abd pain	[] []	Back pain	[] []	Syncope	[] []
Epistaxis	[] []	BM changes	[] []	Heme: bleeding	[] []	Psych: anxiety	[] []
Sinus Sx	[] []	N/V	[] []	Bruising	[] []	Depression	[] []
Hearing loss	[] []	Diarrhea	[] []	Lymph: swelling	[] []	Hallucinations	[] []
Tinnitus	[] []	Heartburn	[] []	Endo: polyuria	[] []	All/Imm: hayfever	[] []
						Runny nose	[] []

Other ROS: _____

Past Medical History:
_____
_____
_____
_____
_____
_____
_____

Past Surgical History:
_____
_____
_____
_____

Family History:
_____
_____
_____

Social History:
_____

Cigs: [] No Yes [] → Pack yrs _____
ETOH [] No Yes [] → Amount? _____
Illicits [] No Yes [] → Type? _____
Allergies: [] NKDA _____
Medications:
_____
_____
_____
_____
_____
_____
_____
_____
_____
_____

[] All other ROS reviewed and were NEGATIVE

Physical Exam T _____ BP _____ HR _____ Wt _____ (lbs) Ht _____ (in) BMI _____

Eyes		**ENT** External		**Neck** External	
Eyes	[] nl conjunctiva & lids	ENT External	[] no scars, lesions, masses	Neck External	[] no tracheal deviation
Pupils	[] equal, round, & reactive	Otoscopic	[] nl canals, TM	Palpation	[] no masses
Fundus	[] nl discs and vessels	Hearing	[] nl hearing	Thyroid	[] no enlargement
Vision	[] acuity & gross fields intact	Oropharynx	[] nl teeth, tongue, pharynx	Abnormals:	
Abnormals:		Abnormals:			

GI Palpation	[] no masses or tenderness	**Resp** Effort	[] nl w/o retractions	**Skin**	[] no rashes, or lesions
	[] no hep/splenomegaly	Percussion	[] no dullness	Chest	[] nl breast, no d/c
Ausculation	[] nl bowel sounds	Palpation	[] no fremitus	Lymph nodes	[] no axillary, inguinal, cervical or submandibular LAD
Percussion	[] no dullness	Ausculation	[] CTA w/o W, R, or R	GU	[] nl male/female exam
Anus/rectum	[] no abnormality or masses	Abnormals:		Psych	[] nl cognition
	[] heme negative stool			Abnormals:	
Abnormals:					

CV Palpation	[] PMI nondisplaced	**Neuro** Orientation	[] AAO x 3
Auscultation	[] no murmur, gallop, or rub	Cranial nerves	[] CN II-XII intact
Carotids	[] nl intensity w/o bruit	Sensory	[] nl sensation
JVD	[] no jugulovenous distention	Reflexes	[] 2+ & symmetrical
Pulses	[] 2+/= femoral & pedal pulses	Abnormals:	
Edema	[] no pedal edema		
Abnormals			

Musculoskeletal	Inspection	ROM	Strength	Tone (✓ if normal)	Abnormals:	**Other:**
Upper extremity	[]	[]	[]	[]		
Lower extremity	[]	[]	[]	[]		
Gait	[] nl gait and FROM					

Labs:

Assessment & Plan:
_____
_____
_____
_____
_____
_____
_____
_____
_____
_____
_____
_____

Clinical Rotation_____   Date: _____

Chief Complaint:
_____

History of Present Illness:
_____
_____
_____
_____
_____

Review of Systems:

	Yes	No		Yes	No		Yes	No		Yes	No
General: fatigue	[]	[]	CV: chest pain	[]	[]	Bloody stool	[]	[]	Polydypsia	[]	[]
Weight loss	[]	[]	Edema	[]	[]	GU: dysuria	[]	[]	Polyphagia	[]	[]
Fever	[]	[]	PND	[]	[]	Frequency	[]	[]	Polyphagia	[]	[]
Chills	[]	[]	Orthopnea	[]	[]	Hematuria	[]	[]	Temp int	[]	[]
Night sweats	[]	[]	Palpitations	[]	[]	Discharge	[]	[]	Derm: rash	[]	[]
Eye: vision change	[]	[]	Claudication	[]	[]	Flank pain	[]	[]	Pruritis	[]	[]
Pain	[]	[]	Resp: cough	[]	[]	MS: arthralgia	[]	[]	Neuro: weakness	[]	[]
Redness	[]	[]	SOB	[]	[]	Arthritis	[]	[]	Seizures	[]	[]
ENT: headaches	[]	[]	Wheezing	[]	[]	Joint swelling	[]	[]	Parasthesias	[]	[]
Hoarseness	[]	[]	Hemoptysis	[]	[]	Myalgias	[]	[]	Tremors	[]	[]
Sore throat	[]	[]	GI: abd pain	[]	[]	Back pain	[]	[]	Syncope	[]	[]
Epistaxis	[]	[]	BM changes	[]	[]	Heme: bleeding	[]	[]	Psych: anxiety	[]	[]
Sinus Sx	[]	[]	N/V	[]	[]	Bruising	[]	[]	Depression	[]	[]
Hearing loss	[]	[]	Diarrhea	[]	[]	Lymph: swelling	[]	[]	Hallucinations	[]	[]
Tinnitus	[]	[]	Heartburn	[]	[]	Endo: polyuria	[]	[]	All/Imm: hayfever	[]	[]
									Runny nose	[]	[]

Other ROS: _____

Past Medical History:
_____
_____
_____
_____
_____
_____

Past Surgical History:
_____
_____
_____
_____

Family History:
_____
_____

[] All other ROS reviewed and were NEGATIVE

Social History:
_____

Cigs: [] No Yes [] → Pack yrs _____
ETOH [] No Yes [] → Amount? _____
Illicits [] No Yes [] → Type?   _____
Allergies: [] NKDA _____
Medications:
_____
_____
_____
_____
_____
_____
_____
_____
_____
_____
_____

Physical Exam T _____ BP _____ HR _____ Wt _____(lbs) Ht _____(in) BMI _____		
Eyes [] nl conjunctiva & lids	**ENT** External [] no scars, lesions, masses	**Neck** External [] no tracheal deviation
Pupils [] equal, round, & reactive	Otoscopic [] nl canals, TM	Palpation [] no masses
Fundus [] nl discs and vessels	Hearing [] nl hearing	Thyroid [] no enlargement
Vision [] acuity & gross fields intact	Oropharynx [] nl teeth, tongue, pharynx	Abnormals:
Abnormals:	Abnormals:	
GI Palpation [] no masses or tenderness [] no hep/splenomegaly	**Resp** Effort [] nl w/o retractions	**Skin** [] no rashes, or lesions
Ausculation [] nl bowel sounds	Percussion [] no dullness	Chest [] nl breast, no d/c
Percussion [] no dullness	Palpation [] no fremitus	Lymph nodes [] no axillary, inguinal, cervical or submandibular LAD
Anus/rectum [] no abnormality or masses [] heme negative stool	Ausculation [] CTA w/o W, R, or R	GU [] nl male/female exam
Abnormals:	Abnormals:	Psych [] nl cognition
CV Palpation [] PMI nondisplaced	**Neuro** Orientation [] AAO x 3	Abnormals:
Auscultation [] no murmur, gallop, or rub	Cranial nerves [] CN II-XII intact	
Carotids [] nl intensity w/o bruit	Sensory [] nl sensation	
JVD [] no jugulovenous distention	Reflexes [] 2+ & symmetrical	
Pulses [] 2+/= femoral & pedal pulses	Abnormals:	
Edema [] no pedal edema		
Abnormals		

Musculoskeletal Inspection ROM Strength Tone (✓ if normal) Abnormals: **Other:**

	Inspection	ROM	Strength	Tone
Upper extremity	[]	[]	[]	[]
Lower extremity	[]	[]	[]	[]

Gait [] nl gait and FROM

Labs:

Assessment & Plan:

_____
_____
_____
_____
_____
_____
_____
_____
_____
_____

Clinical Rotation_____   Date: _____

Chief Complaint:
_____

History of Present Illness:
_____
_____
_____
_____
_____

Review of Systems:

	Yes	No		Yes	No		Yes	No		Yes	No
General: fatigue	[]	[]	CV: chest pain	[]	[]	Bloody stool	[]	[]	Polydypsia	[]	[]
Weight loss	[]	[]	Edema	[]	[]	GU: dysuria	[]	[]	Polyphagia	[]	[]
Fever	[]	[]	PND	[]	[]	Frequency	[]	[]	Polyphagia	[]	[]
Chills	[]	[]	Orthopnea	[]	[]	Hematuria	[]	[]	Temp int	[]	[]
Night sweats	[]	[]	Palpitations	[]	[]	Discharge	[]	[]	Derm: rash	[]	[]
Eye: vision change	[]	[]	Claudication	[]	[]	Flank pain	[]	[]	Pruritis	[]	[]
Pain	[]	[]	Resp: cough	[]	[]	MS: arthralgia	[]	[]	Neuro: weakness	[]	[]
Redness	[]	[]	SOB	[]	[]	Arthritis	[]	[]	Seizures	[]	[]
ENT: headaches	[]	[]	Wheezing	[]	[]	Joint swelling	[]	[]	Parasthesias	[]	[]
Hoarseness	[]	[]	Hemoptysis	[]	[]	Myalgias	[]	[]	Tremors	[]	[]
Sore throat	[]	[]	GI: abd pain	[]	[]	Back pain	[]	[]	Syncope	[]	[]
Epistaxis	[]	[]	BM changes	[]	[]	Heme: bleeding	[]	[]	Psych: anxiety	[]	[]
Sinus Sx	[]	[]	N/V	[]	[]	Bruising	[]	[]	Depression	[]	[]
Hearing loss	[]	[]	Diarrhea	[]	[]	Lymph: swelling	[]	[]	Hallucinations	[]	[]
Tinnitus	[]	[]	Heartburn	[]	[]	Endo: polyuria	[]	[]	All/Imm: hayfever	[]	[]
									Runny nose	[]	[]

Other ROS: _____

Past Medical History:
_____
_____
_____
_____
_____
_____

Past Surgical History:
_____
_____
_____
_____

Family History:
_____

[] All other ROS reviewed and were NEGATIVE

Social History:
_____

Cigs: [] No Yes [] → Pack yrs _____
ETOH [] No Yes [] → Amount? _____
Illicits [] No Yes [] → Type? _____
Allergies: [] NKDA _____
Medications:
_____
_____
_____
_____
_____
_____
_____
_____
_____
_____
_____

Physical Exam   T _____   BP _____   HR _____   Wt _____ (lbs)   Ht _____ (in)   BMI _____

Eyes	[] nl conjunctiva & lids	**ENT** External	[] no scars, lesions, masses	**Neck** External	[]	no tracheal deviation
Pupils	[] equal, round, & reactive	Otoscopic	[] nl canals, TM	Palpation	[]	no masses
Fundus	[] nl discs and vessels	Hearing	[] nl hearing	Thyroid	[]	no enlargement
Vision	[] acuity & gross fields intact	Oropharynx	[] nl teeth, tongue, pharynx	Abnormals:		
Abnormals:		Abnormals:				

GI Palpation	[] no masses or tenderness [] no hep/splenomegaly	**Resp** Effort	[] nl w/o retractions	**Skin**	[] no rashes, or lesions	
Ausculation	[] nl bowel sounds	Percussion	[] no dullness	Chest	[] nl breast, no d/c	
Percussion	[] no dullness	Palpation	[] no fremitus	Lymph nodes	[] no axillary, inguinal, cervical or submandibular LAD	
Anus/rectum	[] no abnormality or masses [] heme negative stool	Ausculation	[] CTA w/o W, R, or R	GU	[] nl male/female exam	
Abnormals:		Abnormals:		Psych	[] nl cognition	

CV Palpation	[] PMI nondisplaced	**Neuro** Orientation	[] AAO x 3	Abnormals:	
Auscultation	[] no murmur, gallop, or rub	Cranial nerves	[] CN II-XII intact		
Carotids	[] nl intensity w/o bruit	Sensory	[] nl sensation		
JVD	[] no jugulovenous distention	Reflexes	[] 2+ & symmetrical		
Pulses	[] 2+/= femoral & pedal pulses	Abnormals:			
Edema	[] no pedal edema				
Abnormals					

Musculoskeletal   Inspection   ROM   Strength   Tone (✓ if normal)   Abnormals:

	Inspection	ROM	Strength	Tone	Other:
Upper extremity	[]	[]	[]	[]	
Lower extremity	[]	[]	[]	[]	
Gait	[] nl gait and FROM				

Labs:

Assessment & Plan:

Clinical Rotation_____   Date: _____

Chief Complaint:

_____

History of Present Illness:

_____
_____
_____
_____
_____

Review of Systems:

	Yes	No		Yes	No		Yes	No		Yes	No
General: fatigue	[]	[]	CV: chest pain	[]	[]	Bloody stool	[]	[]	Polydypsia	[]	[]
Weight loss	[]	[]	Edema	[]	[]	GU: dysuria	[]	[]	Polyphagia	[]	[]
Fever	[]	[]	PND	[]	[]	Frequency	[]	[]	Polyphagia	[]	[]
Chills	[]	[]	Orthopnea	[]	[]	Hematuria	[]	[]	Temp int	[]	[]
Night sweats	[]	[]	Palpitations	[]	[]	Discharge	[]	[]	Derm: rash	[]	[]
Eye: vision change	[]	[]	Claudication	[]	[]	Flank pain	[]	[]	Pruritis	[]	[]
Pain	[]	[]	Resp: cough	[]	[]	MS: arthralgia	[]	[]	Neuro: weakness	[]	[]
Redness	[]	[]	SOB	[]	[]	Arthritis	[]	[]	Seizures	[]	[]
ENT: headaches	[]	[]	Wheezing	[]	[]	Joint swelling	[]	[]	Parasthesias	[]	[]
Hoarseness	[]	[]	Hemoptysis	[]	[]	Myalgias	[]	[]	Tremors	[]	[]
Sore throat	[]	[]	GI: abd pain	[]	[]	Back pain	[]	[]	Syncope	[]	[]
Epistaxis	[]	[]	BM changes	[]	[]	Heme: bleeding	[]	[]	Psych: anxiety	[]	[]
Sinus Sx	[]	[]	N/V	[]	[]	Bruising	[]	[]	Depression	[]	[]
Hearing loss	[]	[]	Diarrhea	[]	[]	Lymph: swelling	[]	[]	Hallucinations	[]	[]
Tinnitus	[]	[]	Heartburn	[]	[]	Endo: polyuria	[]	[]	All/Imm: hayfever	[]	[]
									Runny nose	[]	[]

Other ROS: _____

Past Medical History:

_____
_____
_____
_____
_____
_____

Past Surgical History:

_____
_____
_____
_____

Family History:

_____
_____

[] All other ROS reviewed and were NEGATIVE

Social History:

_____

Cigs: [] No Yes [] → Pack yrs _____
ETOH [] No Yes [] → Amount? _____
Illicits [] No Yes [] → Type? _____
Allergies: [] NKDA _____
Medications:

_____
_____
_____
_____
_____
_____
_____
_____

Physical Exam   T _____   BP _____   HR _____   Wt _____(lbs)   Ht _____(in)   BMI _____

Eyes [] nl conjunctiva & lids	**ENT** External [] no scars, lesions, masses	**Neck** External [] no tracheal deviation
Pupils [] equal, round, & reactive	Otoscopic [] nl canals, TM	Palpation [] no masses
Fundus [] nl discs and vessels	Hearing [] nl hearing	Thyroid [] no enlargement
Vision [] acuity & gross fields intact	Oropharynx [] nl teeth, tongue, pharynx	Abnormals:
Abnormals:	Abnormals:	
GI Palpation [] no masses or tenderness [] no hep/splenomegaly	**Resp** Effort [] nl w/o retractions	**Skin** [] no rashes, or lesions
Ausculation [] nl bowel sounds	Percussion [] no dullness	Chest [] nl breast, no d/c
Percussion [] no dullness	Palpation [] no fremitus	Lymph nodes [] no axillary, inguinal, cervical or submandibular LAD
Anus/rectum [] no abnormality or masses [] heme negative stool	Ausculation [] CTA w/o W, R, or R Abnormals:	GU [] nl male/female exam
Abnormals:		Psych [] nl cognition
CV Palpation [] PMI nondisplaced	**Neuro** Orientation [] AAO x 3	Abnormals:
Auscultation [] no murmur, gallop, or rub	Cranial nerves [] CN II-XII intact	
Carotids [] nl intensity w/o bruit	Sensory [] nl sensation	
JVD [] no jugulovenous distention	Reflexes [] 2+ & symmetrical	
Pulses [] 2+/= femoral & pedal pulses	Abnormals:	
Edema [] no pedal edema		
Abnormals		

Musculoskeletal Inspection ROM Strength Tone (✓ if normal) Abnormals:	**Other:**
Upper extremity [] [] [] [] Lower extremity [] [] [] [] Gait [] nl gait and FROM	

Labs:

Assessment & Plan:

_____
_____
_____
_____
_____
_____
_____
_____
_____
_____

Clinical Rotation_____   Date: _____

Chief Complaint:
_____

History of Present Illness:
_____
_____
_____
_____
_____

Review of Systems:

	Yes	No		Yes	No		Yes	No		Yes	No
General: fatigue	[]	[]	CV: chest pain	[]	[]	Bloody stool	[]	[]	Polydypsia	[]	[]
Weight loss	[]	[]	Edema	[]	[]	GU: dysuria	[]	[]	Polyphagia	[]	[]
Fever	[]	[]	PND	[]	[]	Frequency	[]	[]	Polyphagia	[]	[]
Chills	[]	[]	Orthopnea	[]	[]	Hematuria	[]	[]	Temp int	[]	[]
Night sweats	[]	[]	Palpitations	[]	[]	Discharge	[]	[]	Derm: rash	[]	[]
Eye: vision change	[]	[]	Claudication	[]	[]	Flank pain	[]	[]	Pruritis	[]	[]
Pain	[]	[]	Resp: cough	[]	[]	MS: arthralgia	[]	[]	Neuro: weakness	[]	[]
Redness	[]	[]	SOB	[]	[]	Arthritis	[]	[]	Seizures	[]	[]
ENT: headaches	[]	[]	Wheezing	[]	[]	Joint swelling	[]	[]	Parasthesias	[]	[]
Hoarseness	[]	[]	Hemoptysis	[]	[]	Myalgias	[]	[]	Tremors	[]	[]
Sore throat	[]	[]	GI: abd pain	[]	[]	Back pain	[]	[]	Syncope	[]	[]
Epistaxis	[]	[]	BM changes	[]	[]	Heme: bleeding	[]	[]	Psych: anxiety	[]	[]
Sinus Sx	[]	[]	N/V	[]	[]	Bruising	[]	[]	Depression	[]	[]
Hearing loss	[]	[]	Diarrhea	[]	[]	Lymph: swelling	[]	[]	Hallucinations	[]	[]
Tinnitus	[]	[]	Heartburn	[]	[]	Endo: polyuria	[]	[]	All/Imm: hayfever	[]	[]
									Runny nose	[]	[]

Other ROS: _____

Past Medical History:
_____
_____
_____
_____
_____
_____

Past Surgical History:
_____
_____
_____
_____

Family History:
_____
_____

[] All other ROS reviewed and were NEGATIVE

Social History:
_____

Cigs: [] No Yes [] → Pack yrs _____
ETOH [] No Yes [] → Amount? _____
Illicits [] No Yes [] → Type? _____
Allergies: [] NKDA _____
Medications:
_____
_____
_____
_____
_____
_____
_____
_____

Physical Exam T _____ BP _____ HR _____ Wt _____(lbs) Ht _____(in) BMI _____		
Eyes [] nl conjunctiva & lids	**ENT** External [] no scars, lesions, masses	**Neck** External [] no tracheal deviation
Pupils [] equal, round, & reactive	Otoscopic [] nl canals, TM	Palpation [] no masses
Fundus [] nl discs and vessels	Hearing [] nl hearing	Thyroid [] no enlargement
Vision [] acuity & gross fields intact	Oropharynx [] nl teeth, tongue, pharynx	Abnormals:
Abnormals:	Abnormals:	
GI Palpation [] no masses or tenderness [] no hep/splenomegaly	**Resp** Effort [] nl w/o retractions	**Skin** [] no rashes, or lesions
	Percussion [] no dullness	Chest [] nl breast, no d/c
Ausculation [] nl bowel sounds	Palpation [] no fremitus	Lymph nodes [] no axillary, inguinal, cervical or submandibular LAD
Percussion [] no dullness	Ausculation [] CTA w/o W, R, or R	
Anus/rectum [] no abnormality or masses [] heme negative stool	Abnormals:	GU [] nl male/female exam
Abnormals:		Psych [] nl cognition
CV Palpation [] PMI nondisplaced	**Neuro** Orientation [] AAO x 3	Abnormals:
Auscultation [] no murmur, gallop, or rub	Cranial nerves [] CN II-XII intact	
Carotids [] nl intensity w/o bruit	Sensory [] nl sensation	
JVD [] no jugulovenous distention	Reflexes [] 2+ & symmetrical	
Pulses [] 2+/= femoral & pedal pulses	Abnormals:	
Edema [] no pedal edema		
Abnormals		

Musculoskeletal	Inspection	ROM	Strength	Tone (✓ if normal)	Abnormals:	Other:
Upper extremity	[]	[]	[]	[]		
Lower extremity	[]	[]	[]	[]		
Gait	[] nl gait and FROM					

Labs:

Assessment & Plan:
_____
_____
_____
_____
_____
_____
_____
_____
_____
_____
_____

Clinical Rotation_____   Date: _____

Chief Complaint:
_____

History of Present Illness:
_____
_____
_____
_____
_____

Review of Systems:

	Yes	No		Yes	No		Yes	No		Yes	No
General: fatigue	[]	[]	CV: chest pain	[]	[]	Bloody stool	[]	[]	Polydypsia	[]	[]
Weight loss	[]	[]	Edema	[]	[]	GU: dysuria	[]	[]	Polyphagia	[]	[]
Fever	[]	[]	PND	[]	[]	Frequency	[]	[]	Polyphagia	[]	[]
Chills	[]	[]	Orthopnea	[]	[]	Hematuria	[]	[]	Temp int	[]	[]
Night sweats	[]	[]	Palpitations	[]	[]	Discharge	[]	[]	Derm: rash	[]	[]
Eye: vision change	[]	[]	Claudication	[]	[]	Flank pain	[]	[]	Pruritis	[]	[]
Pain	[]	[]	Resp: cough	[]	[]	MS: arthralgia	[]	[]	Neuro: weakness	[]	[]
Redness	[]	[]	SOB	[]	[]	Arthritis	[]	[]	Seizures	[]	[]
ENT: headaches	[]	[]	Wheezing	[]	[]	Joint swelling	[]	[]	Parasthesias	[]	[]
Hoarseness	[]	[]	Hemoptysis	[]	[]	Myalgias	[]	[]	Tremors	[]	[]
Sore throat	[]	[]	GI: abd pain	[]	[]	Back pain	[]	[]	Syncope	[]	[]
Epistaxis	[]	[]	BM changes	[]	[]	Heme: bleeding	[]	[]	Psych: anxiety	[]	[]
Sinus Sx	[]	[]	N/V	[]	[]	Bruising	[]	[]	Depression	[]	[]
Hearing loss	[]	[]	Diarrhea	[]	[]	Lymph: swelling	[]	[]	Hallucinations	[]	[]
Tinnitus	[]	[]	Heartburn	[]	[]	Endo: polyuria	[]	[]	All/Imm: hayfever	[]	[]
									Runny nose	[]	[]

Other ROS: _____

Past Medical History:
_____
_____
_____
_____
_____
_____

Past Surgical History:
_____
_____
_____

Family History:
_____
_____

[] All other ROS reviewed and were NEGATIVE

Social History:
_____

Cigs: [] No Yes [] → Pack yrs _____
ETOH [] No Yes [] → Amount? _____
Illicits [] No Yes [] → Type? _____
Allergies: [] NKDA _____
Medications:
_____
_____
_____
_____
_____
_____
_____
_____

Physical Exam T _____ BP _____ HR _____ Wt _____ (lbs) Ht _____ (in) BMI _____		
Eyes [] nl conjunctiva & lids	**ENT** External [] no scars, lesions, masses	**Neck** External [] no tracheal deviation
Pupils [] equal, round, & reactive	Otoscopic [] nl canals, TM	Palpation [] no masses
Fundus [] nl discs and vessels	Hearing [] nl hearing	Thyroid [] no enlargement
Vision [] acuity & gross fields intact	Oropharynx [] nl teeth, tongue, pharynx	Abnormals:
Abnormals:	Abnormals:	
GI Palpation [] no masses or tenderness [] no hep/splenomegaly	**Resp** Effort [] nl w/o retractions	**Skin** [] no rashes, or lesions
	Percussion [] no dullness	Chest [] nl breast, no d/c
Ausculation [] nl bowel sounds	Palpation [] no fremitus	Lymph nodes [] no axillary, inguinal,
Percussion [] no dullness	Ausculation [] CTA w/o W, R, or R	cervical or submandibular LAD
Anus/rectum [] no abnormality or masses [] heme negative stool	Abnormals:	GU [] nl male/female exam
Abnormals:		Psych [] nl cognition
CV Palpation [] PMI nondisplaced	**Neuro** Orientation [] AAO x 3	Abnormals:
Auscultation [] no murmur, gallop, or rub	Cranial nerves [] CN II-XII intact	
Carotids [] nl intensity w/o bruit	Sensory [] nl sensation	
JVD [] no jugulovenous distention	Reflexes [] 2+ & symmetrical	
Pulses [] 2+/= femoral & pedal pulses	Abnormals:	
Edema [] no pedal edema		
Abnormals		
Musculoskeletal Inspection ROM Strength Tone (✓ if normal) Abnormals:		**Other:**
Upper extremity [] [] [] [] Lower extremity [] [] [] []		
Gait [] nl gait and FROM		

Labs:

Assessment & Plan:

_____
_____
_____
_____
_____
_____
_____
_____
_____
_____
_____
_____

Clinical Rotation_____   Date: _____

Chief Complaint:

_____

History of Present Illness:

_____
_____
_____
_____
_____

Review of Systems:

	Yes	No		Yes	No		Yes	No		Yes	No
General: fatigue	[]	[]	CV: chest pain	[]	[]	Bloody stool	[]	[]	Polydypsia	[]	[]
Weight loss	[]	[]	Edema	[]	[]	GU: dysuria	[]	[]	Polyphagia	[]	[]
Fever	[]	[]	PND	[]	[]	Frequency	[]	[]	Polyphagia	[]	[]
Chills	[]	[]	Orthopnea	[]	[]	Hematuria	[]	[]	Temp int	[]	[]
Night sweats	[]	[]	Palpitations	[]	[]	Discharge	[]	[]	Derm: rash	[]	[]
Eye: vision change	[]	[]	Claudication	[]	[]	Flank pain	[]	[]	Pruritis	[]	[]
Pain	[]	[]	Resp: cough	[]	[]	MS: arthralgia	[]	[]	Neuro: weakness	[]	[]
Redness	[]	[]	SOB	[]	[]	Arthritis	[]	[]	Seizures	[]	[]
ENT: headaches	[]	[]	Wheezing	[]	[]	Joint swelling	[]	[]	Parasthesias	[]	[]
Hoarseness	[]	[]	Hemoptysis	[]	[]	Myalgias	[]	[]	Tremors	[]	[]
Sore throat	[]	[]	GI: abd pain	[]	[]	Back pain	[]	[]	Syncope	[]	[]
Epistaxis	[]	[]	BM changes	[]	[]	Heme: bleeding	[]	[]	Psych: anxiety	[]	[]
Sinus Sx	[]	[]	N/V	[]	[]	Bruising	[]	[]	Depression	[]	[]
Hearing loss	[]	[]	Diarrhea	[]	[]	Lymph: swelling	[]	[]	Hallucinations	[]	[]
Tinnitus	[]	[]	Heartburn	[]	[]	Endo: polyuria	[]	[]	All/Imm: hayfever	[]	[]
									Runny nose	[]	[]

Other ROS: _____

Past Medical History:

_____
_____
_____
_____
_____
_____

Past Surgical History:

_____
_____
_____

Family History:

_____
_____

[] All other ROS reviewed and were NEGATIVE

Social History:

_____
_____

Cigs: [] No Yes [] → Pack yrs _____
ETOH [] No Yes [] → Amount? _____
Illicits [] No Yes [] → Type? _____
Allergies: [] NKDA _____
Medications:

_____
_____
_____
_____
_____
_____
_____
_____
_____
_____
_____
_____

Physical Exam T _____ BP _____ HR _____ Wt _____ (lbs) Ht _____ (in) BMI _____		
Eyes [] nl conjunctiva & lids	**ENT** External [] no scars, lesions, masses	**Neck** External [] no tracheal deviation
Pupils [] equal, round, & reactive	Otoscopic [] nl canals, TM	Palpation [] no masses
Fundus [] nl discs and vessels	Hearing [] nl hearing	Thyroid [] no enlargement
Vision [] acuity & gross fields intact	Oropharynx [] nl teeth, tongue, pharynx	Abnormals:
Abnormals:	Abnormals:	
GI Palpation [] no masses or tenderness [] no hep/splenomegaly	**Resp** Effort [] nl w/o retractions	**Skin** [] no rashes, or lesions
Ausculation [] nl bowel sounds	Percussion [] no dullness	Chest [] nl breast, no d/c
Percussion [] no dullness	Palpation [] no fremitus	Lymph nodes [] no axillary, inguinal, cervical or submandibular LAD
Anus/rectum [] no abnormality or masses [] heme negative stool	Ausculation [] CTA w/o W, R, or R	GU [] nl male/female exam
Abnormals:	Abnormals:	Psych [] nl cognition
CV Palpation [] PMI nondisplaced	**Neuro** Orientation [] AAO x 3	Abnormals:
Auscultation [] no murmur, gallop, or rub	Cranial nerves [] CN II-XII intact	
Carotids [] nl intensity w/o bruit	Sensory [] nl sensation	
JVD [] no jugulovenous distention	Reflexes [] 2+ & symmetrical	
Pulses [] 2+/= femoral & pedal pulses	Abnormals:	
Edema [] no pedal edema		
Abnormals		
Musculoskeletal Inspection ROM Strength Tone (✓ if normal) Abnormals:		**Other:**
Upper extremity [] [] [] [] Lower extremity [] [] [] []		
Gait [] nl gait and FROM		

Labs:

Assessment & Plan:

_____
_____
_____
_____
_____
_____
_____
_____
_____
_____
_____
_____

Clinical Rotation_____   Date: _____

Chief Complaint:
_____

History of Present Illness:
_____
_____
_____
_____
_____

Review of Systems:

	Yes	No		Yes	No		Yes	No		Yes	No
General: fatigue	[]	[]	CV: chest pain	[]	[]	Bloody stool	[]	[]	Polydypsia	[]	[]
Weight loss	[]	[]	Edema	[]	[]	GU: dysuria	[]	[]	Polyphagia	[]	[]
Fever	[]	[]	PND	[]	[]	Frequency	[]	[]	Polyphagia	[]	[]
Chills	[]	[]	Orthopnea	[]	[]	Hematuria	[]	[]	Temp int	[]	[]
Night sweats	[]	[]	Palpitations	[]	[]	Discharge	[]	[]	Derm: rash	[]	[]
Eye: vision change	[]	[]	Claudication	[]	[]	Flank pain	[]	[]	Pruritis	[]	[]
Pain	[]	[]	Resp: cough	[]	[]	MS: arthralgia	[]	[]	Neuro: weakness	[]	[]
Redness	[]	[]	SOB	[]	[]	Arthritis	[]	[]	Seizures	[]	[]
ENT: headaches	[]	[]	Wheezing	[]	[]	Joint swelling	[]	[]	Parasthesias	[]	[]
Hoarseness	[]	[]	Hemoptysis	[]	[]	Myalgias	[]	[]	Tremors	[]	[]
Sore throat	[]	[]	GI: abd pain	[]	[]	Back pain	[]	[]	Syncope	[]	[]
Epistaxis	[]	[]	BM changes	[]	[]	Heme: bleeding	[]	[]	Psych: anxiety	[]	[]
Sinus Sx	[]	[]	N/V	[]	[]	Bruising	[]	[]	Depression	[]	[]
Hearing loss	[]	[]	Diarrhea	[]	[]	Lymph: swelling	[]	[]	Hallucinations	[]	[]
Tinnitus	[]	[]	Heartburn	[]	[]	Endo: polyuria	[]	[]	All/Imm: hayfever	[]	[]
									Runny nose	[]	[]

Other ROS: _____

Past Medical History:
_____
_____
_____
_____
_____
_____

Past Surgical History:
_____
_____
_____
_____

Family History:
_____
_____

Social History:
_____
_____

Cigs: [] No Yes [] → Pack yrs _____
ETOH [] No Yes [] → Amount? _____
Illicits [] No Yes [] → Type? _____
Allergies: [] NKDA _____
Medications:
_____
_____
_____
_____
_____
_____
_____
_____

[] All other ROS reviewed and were NEGATIVE

Physical Exam T _____ BP _____ HR _____ Wt _____(lbs) Ht _____(in) BMI _____		

Eyes		**ENT** External	[] no scars, lesions, masses	**Neck** External	[] no tracheal deviation
Eyes	[] nl conjunctiva & lids	ENT External	[] no scars, lesions, masses	Neck External	[] no tracheal deviation
Pupils	[] equal, round, & reactive	Otoscopic	[] nl canals, TM	Palpation	[] no masses
Fundus	[] nl discs and vessels	Hearing	[] nl hearing	Thyroid	[] no enlargement
Vision	[] acuity & gross fields intact	Oropharynx	[] nl teeth, tongue, pharynx	Abnormals:	
Abnormals:		Abnormals:			
GI Palpation	[] no masses or tenderness [] no hep/splenomegaly	**Resp** Effort	[] nl w/o retractions	**Skin**	[] no rashes, or lesions
		Percussion	[] no dullness	Chest	[] nl breast, no d/c
Ausculation	[] nl bowel sounds	Palpation	[] no fremitus	Lymph nodes	[] no axillary, inguinal, cervical or submandibular LAD
Percussion	[] no dullness	Ausculation	[] CTA w/o W, R, or R		
Anus/rectum	[] no abnormality or masses [] heme negative stool	Abnormals:		GU	[] nl male/female exam
Abnormals:				Psych	[] nl cognition
CV Palpation	[] PMI nondisplaced	**Neuro** Orientation	[] AAO x 3	Abnormals:	
Auscultation	[] no murmur, gallop, or rub	Cranial nerves	[] CN II-XII intact		
Carotids	[] nl intensity w/o bruit	Sensory	[] nl sensation		
JVD	[] no jugulovenous distention	Reflexes	[] 2+ & symmetrical		
Pulses	[] 2+/= femoral & pedal pulses	Abnormals:			
Edema	[] no pedal edema				
Abnormals					

Musculoskeletal Inspection ROM Strength Tone (✓ if normal) Abnormals:	**Other:**
Upper extremity [] [] [] []	
Lower extremity [] [] [] []	
Gait [] nl gait and FROM	

Labs:

Assessment & Plan:

_____
_____
_____
_____
_____
_____
_____
_____
_____
_____
_____

Clinical Rotation_____   Date: _____

Chief Complaint:
_____

History of Present Illness:
_____
_____
_____
_____
_____

Review of Systems:

	Yes	No		Yes	No		Yes	No		Yes	No
General: fatigue	[]	[]	CV: chest pain	[]	[]	Bloody stool	[]	[]	Polydypsia	[]	[]
Weight loss	[]	[]	Edema	[]	[]	GU: dysuria	[]	[]	Polyphagia	[]	[]
Fever	[]	[]	PND	[]	[]	Frequency	[]	[]	Polyphagia	[]	[]
Chills	[]	[]	Orthopnea	[]	[]	Hematuria	[]	[]	Temp int	[]	[]
Night sweats	[]	[]	Palpitations	[]	[]	Discharge	[]	[]	Derm: rash	[]	[]
Eye: vision change	[]	[]	Claudication	[]	[]	Flank pain	[]	[]	Pruritis	[]	[]
Pain	[]	[]	Resp: cough	[]	[]	MS: arthralgia	[]	[]	Neuro: weakness	[]	[]
Redness	[]	[]	SOB	[]	[]	Arthritis	[]	[]	Seizures	[]	[]
ENT: headaches	[]	[]	Wheezing	[]	[]	Joint swelling	[]	[]	Parasthesias	[]	[]
Hoarseness	[]	[]	Hemoptysis	[]	[]	Myalgias	[]	[]	Tremors	[]	[]
Sore throat	[]	[]	GI: abd pain	[]	[]	Back pain	[]	[]	Syncope	[]	[]
Epistaxis	[]	[]	BM changes	[]	[]	Heme: bleeding	[]	[]	Psych: anxiety	[]	[]
Sinus Sx	[]	[]	N/V	[]	[]	Bruising	[]	[]	Depression	[]	[]
Hearing loss	[]	[]	Diarrhea	[]	[]	Lymph: swelling	[]	[]	Hallucinations	[]	[]
Tinnitus	[]	[]	Heartburn	[]	[]	Endo: polyuria	[]	[]	All/Imm: hayfever	[]	[]
									Runny nose	[]	[]

Other ROS: _____

Past Medical History:
_____
_____
_____
_____
_____
_____

Social History:
_____

Cigs: [] No Yes [] → Pack yrs _____
ETOH [] No Yes [] → Amount? _____
Illicits [] No Yes [] → Type? _____
Allergies: [] NKDA _____
Medications:

Past Surgical History:
_____
_____
_____
_____

Family History:
_____
_____
_____
_____

[] All other ROS reviewed and were NEGATIVE

Physical Exam T _____ BP _____ HR _____ Wt _____ (lbs) Ht _____ (in) BMI _____

Eyes	[] nl conjunctiva & lids	**ENT** External	[] no scars, lesions, masses	**Neck** External	[] no tracheal deviation
Pupils	[] equal, round, & reactive	Otoscopic	[] nl canals, TM	Palpation	[] no masses
Fundus	[] nl discs and vessels	Hearing	[] nl hearing	Thyroid	[] no enlargement
Vision	[] acuity & gross fields intact	Oropharynx	[] nl teeth, tongue, pharynx	Abnormals:	
Abnormals:		Abnormals:			

GI Palpation	[] no masses or tenderness [] no hep/splenomegaly	**Resp** Effort	[] nl w/o retractions	**Skin**	[] no rashes, or lesions
		Percussion	[] no dullness	Chest	[] nl breast, no d/c
Ausculation	[] nl bowel sounds	Palpation	[] no fremitus	Lymph nodes	[] no axillary, inguinal, cervical or submandibular LAD
Percussion	[] no dullness	Ausculation	[] CTA w/o W, R, or R		
Anus/rectum	[] no abnormality or masses [] heme negative stool	Abnormals:		GU	[] nl male/female exam
Abnormals:				Psych	[] nl cognition

CV Palpation	[] PMI nondisplaced	**Neuro** Orientation	[] AAO x 3	Abnormals:	
Auscultation	[] no murmur, gallop, or rub	Cranial nerves	[] CN II-XII intact		
Carotids	[] nl intensity w/o bruit	Sensory	[] nl sensation		
JVD	[] no jugulovenous distention	Reflexes	[] 2+ & symmetrical		
Pulses	[] 2+/= femoral & pedal pulses	Abnormals:			
Edema	[] no pedal edema				
Abnormals					

Musculoskeletal	Inspection	ROM	Strength	Tone	(✓ if normal) Abnormals:	**Other:**
Upper extremity	[]	[]	[]	[]		
Lower extremity	[]	[]	[]	[]		
Gait	[] nl gait and FROM					

Labs:

Assessment & Plan:

_____
_____
_____
_____
_____
_____
_____
_____
_____
_____
_____

Clinical Rotation_____　　　　　　　　**Date:** _____

Chief Complaint:
_____

History of Present Illness:
_____
_____
_____
_____
_____

Review of Systems:

	Yes No		Yes No		Yes No		Yes No
General: fatigue	[] []	CV: chest pain	[] []	Bloody stool	[] []	Polydypsia	[] []
Weight loss	[] []	Edema	[] []	GU: dysuria	[] []	Polyphagia	[] []
Fever	[] []	PND	[] []	Frequency	[] []	Polyphagia	[] []
Chills	[] []	Orthopnea	[] []	Hematuria	[] []	Temp int	[] []
Night sweats	[] []	Palpitations	[] []	Discharge	[] []	Derm: rash	[] []
Eye: vision change	[] []	Claudication	[] []	Flank pain	[] []	Pruritis	[] []
Pain	[] []	Resp: cough	[] []	MS: arthralgia	[] []	Neuro: weakness	[] []
Redness	[] []	SOB	[] []	Arthritis	[] []	Seizures	[] []
ENT: headaches	[] []	Wheezing	[] []	Joint swelling	[] []	Parasthesias	[] []
Hoarseness	[] []	Hemoptysis	[] []	Myalgias	[] []	Tremors	[] []
Sore throat	[] []	GI: abd pain	[] []	Back pain	[] []	Syncope	[] []
Epistaxis	[] []	BM changes	[] []	Heme: bleeding	[] []	Psych: anxiety	[] []
Sinus Sx	[] []	N/V	[] []	Bruising	[] []	Depression	[] []
Hearing loss	[] []	Diarrhea	[] []	Lymph: swelling	[] []	Hallucinations	[] []
Tinnitus	[] []	Heartburn	[] []	Endo: polyuria	[] []	All/Imm: hayfever	[] []
						Runny nose	[] []

Other ROS: _____

Past Medical History:
_____
_____
_____
_____
_____
_____

Past Surgical History:
_____
_____
_____
_____

Family History:
_____
_____
_____

Social History:
_____

Cigs: [] No Yes [] → Pack yrs _____
ETOH [] No Yes [] → Amount? _____
Illicits [] No Yes [] → Type? _____
Allergies: [] NKDA _____
Medications:
_____
_____
_____
_____
_____
_____
_____
_____
_____
_____

[ ] All other ROS reviewed and were NEGATIVE

Physical Exam T _____ BP _____	HR _____ Wt _____(lbs) Ht _____(in) BMI _____	
Eyes [] nl conjunctiva & lids	**ENT** External [] no scars, lesions, masses	**Neck** External [] no tracheal deviation
Pupils [] equal, round, & reactive	Otoscopic [] nl canals, TM	Palpation [] no masses
Fundus [] nl discs and vessels	Hearing [] nl hearing	Thyroid [] no enlargement
Vision [] acuity & gross fields intact	Oropharynx [] nl teeth, tongue, pharynx	Abnormals:
Abnormals:	Abnormals:	
GI Palpation [] no masses or tenderness [] no hep/splenomegaly	**Resp** Effort [] nl w/o retractions	**Skin** [] no rashes, or lesions
Ausculation [] nl bowel sounds	Percussion [] no dullness	Chest [] nl breast, no d/c
Percussion [] no dullness	Palpation [] no fremitus	Lymph nodes [] no axillary, inguinal, cervical or submandibular LAD
Anus/rectum [] no abnormality or masses [] heme negative stool	Ausculation [] CTA w/o W, R, or R Abnormals:	GU [] nl male/female exam
Abnormals:		Psych [] nl cognition
CV Palpation [] PMI nondisplaced	**Neuro** Orientation [] AAO x 3	Abnormals:
Auscultation [] no murmur, gallop, or rub	Cranial nerves [] CN II-XII intact	
Carotids [] nl intensity w/o bruit	Sensory [] nl sensation	
JVD [] no jugulovenous distention	Reflexes [] 2+ & symmetrical	
Pulses [] 2+/= femoral & pedal pulses	Abnormals:	
Edema [] no pedal edema		
Abnormals		
Musculoskeletal Inspection ROM Strength Tone (✔ if normal) Abnormals:		**Other:**
Upper extremity [] [] [] []		
Lower extremity [] [] [] []		
Gait [] nl gait and FROM		

Labs:

Assessment & Plan:

_____
_____
_____
_____
_____
_____
_____
_____
_____
_____
_____

Clinical Rotation_____   Date: _____

Chief Complaint:
_____

History of Present Illness:
_____
_____
_____
_____
_____

Review of Systems:

	Yes No		Yes No		Yes No		Yes No
General: fatigue	[] []	CV: chest pain	[] []	Bloody stool	[] []	Polydypsia	[] []
Weight loss	[] []	Edema	[] []	GU: dysuria	[] []	Polyphagia	[] []
Fever	[] []	PND	[] []	Frequency	[] []	Polyphagia	[] []
Chills	[] []	Orthopnea	[] []	Hematuria	[] []	Temp int	[] []
Night sweats	[] []	Palpitations	[] []	Discharge	[] []	Derm: rash	[] []
Eye: vision change	[] []	Claudication	[] []	Flank pain	[] []	Pruritis	[] []
Pain	[] []	Resp: cough	[] []	MS: arthralgia	[] []	Neuro: weakness	[] []
Redness	[] []	SOB	[] []	Arthritis	[] []	Seizures	[] []
ENT: headaches	[] []	Wheezing	[] []	Joint swelling	[] []	Parasthesias	[] []
Hoarseness	[] []	Hemoptysis	[] []	Myalgias	[] []	Tremors	[] []
Sore throat	[] []	GI: abd pain	[] []	Back pain	[] []	Syncope	[] []
Epistaxis	[] []	BM changes	[] []	Heme: bleeding	[] []	Psych: anxiety	[] []
Sinus Sx	[] []	N/V	[] []	Bruising	[] []	Depression	[] []
Hearing loss	[] []	Diarrhea	[] []	Lymph: swelling	[] []	Hallucinations	[] []
Tinnitus	[] []	Heartburn	[] []	Endo: polyuria	[] []	All/Imm: hayfever	[] []
						Runny nose	[] []

Other ROS: _____

Past Medical History:
_____
_____
_____
_____
_____
_____
_____

Past Surgical History:
_____
_____
_____
_____

Family History:
_____
_____

[] All other ROS reviewed and were NEGATIVE

Social History:
_____

Cigs: [] No Yes [] → Pack yrs _____
ETOH [] No Yes [] → Amount? _____
Illicits [] No Yes [] → Type? _____
Allergies: [] NKDA _____
Medications:
_____
_____
_____
_____
_____
_____
_____
_____

Physical Exam	T _____	BP _____	HR _____	Wt _____ (lbs)	Ht _____ (in)	BMI _____

Eyes	[] nl conjunctiva & lids	**ENT** External	[] no scars, lesions, masses	**Neck** External	[] no tracheal deviation
Pupils	[] equal, round, & reactive	Otoscopic	[] nl canals, TM	Palpation	[] no masses
Fundus	[] nl discs and vessels	Hearing	[] nl hearing	Thyroid	[] no enlargement
Vision	[] acuity & gross fields intact	Oropharynx	[] nl teeth, tongue, pharynx	Abnormals:	
Abnormals:		Abnormals:			

GI Palpation	[] no masses or tenderness [] no hep/splenomegaly	**Resp** Effort	[] nl w/o retractions	**Skin**	[] no rashes, or lesions
Ausculation	[] nl bowel sounds	Percussion	[] no dullness	Chest	[] nl breast, no d/c
Percussion	[] no dullness	Palpation	[] no fremitus	Lymph nodes	[] no axillary, inguinal, cervical or submandibular LAD
Anus/rectum	[] no abnormality or masses [] heme negative stool	Ausculation	[] CTA w/o W, R, or R	GU	[] nl male/female exam
Abnormals:		Abnormals:		Psych	[] nl cognition

CV Palpation	[] PMI nondisplaced	**Neuro** Orientation	[] AAO x 3	Abnormals:	
Auscultation	[] no murmur, gallop, or rub	Cranial nerves	[] CN II-XII intact		
Carotids	[] nl intensity w/o bruit	Sensory	[] nl sensation		
JVD	[] no jugulovenous distention	Reflexes	[] 2+ & symmetrical		
Pulses	[] 2+/= femoral & pedal pulses	Abnormals:			
Edema	[] no pedal edema				
Abnormals					

Musculoskeletal	Inspection	ROM	Strength	Tone (✓ if normal)	Abnormals:	**Other:**
Upper extremity	[]	[]	[]	[]		
Lower extremity	[]	[]	[]	[]		
Gait	[] nl gait and FROM					

Labs:

Assessment & Plan:

_____
_____
_____
_____
_____
_____
_____
_____
_____
_____
_____

Clinical Rotation_____ Date: _____

Chief Complaint:
_____

History of Present Illness:
_____
_____
_____
_____
_____

Review of Systems:

	Yes	No		Yes	No		Yes	No		Yes	No
General: fatigue	[]	[]	CV: chest pain	[]	[]	Bloody stool	[]	[]	Polydypsia	[]	[]
Weight loss	[]	[]	Edema	[]	[]	GU: dysuria	[]	[]	Polyphagia	[]	[]
Fever	[]	[]	PND	[]	[]	Frequency	[]	[]	Polyphagia	[]	[]
Chills	[]	[]	Orthopnea	[]	[]	Hematuria	[]	[]	Temp int	[]	[]
Night sweats	[]	[]	Palpitations	[]	[]	Discharge	[]	[]	Derm: rash	[]	[]
Eye: vision change	[]	[]	Claudication	[]	[]	Flank pain	[]	[]	Pruritis	[]	[]
Pain	[]	[]	Resp: cough	[]	[]	MS: arthralgia	[]	[]	Neuro: weakness	[]	[]
Redness	[]	[]	SOB	[]	[]	Arthritis	[]	[]	Seizures	[]	[]
ENT: headaches	[]	[]	Wheezing	[]	[]	Joint swelling	[]	[]	Parasthesias	[]	[]
Hoarseness	[]	[]	Hemoptysis	[]	[]	Myalgias	[]	[]	Tremors	[]	[]
Sore throat	[]	[]	GI: abd pain	[]	[]	Back pain	[]	[]	Syncope	[]	[]
Epistaxis	[]	[]	BM changes	[]	[]	Heme: bleeding	[]	[]	Psych: anxiety	[]	[]
Sinus Sx	[]	[]	N/V	[]	[]	Bruising	[]	[]	Depression	[]	[]
Hearing loss	[]	[]	Diarrhea	[]	[]	Lymph: swelling	[]	[]	Hallucinations	[]	[]
Tinnitus	[]	[]	Heartburn	[]	[]	Endo: polyuria	[]	[]	All/Imm: hayfever	[]	[]
									Runny nose	[]	[]

Other ROS: _____

Past Medical History:
_____
_____
_____
_____
_____
_____

Past Surgical History:
_____
_____
_____
_____

Family History:
_____

[] All other ROS reviewed and were NEGATIVE

Social History:
_____

Cigs: [] No Yes [] → Pack yrs _____
ETOH [] No Yes [] → Amount? _____
Illicits [] No Yes [] → Type? _____
Allergies: [] NKDA _____
Medications:
_____
_____
_____
_____
_____
_____
_____
_____
_____
_____

Physical Exam T _____ BP _____ HR _____ Wt _____(lbs) Ht _____(in) BMI _____

Eyes	[] nl conjunctiva & lids	**ENT** External	[] no scars, lesions, masses	**Neck** External	[] no tracheal deviation
Pupils	[] equal, round, & reactive	Otoscopic	[] nl canals, TM	Palpation	[] no masses
Fundus	[] nl discs and vessels	Hearing	[] nl hearing	Thyroid	[] no enlargement
Vision	[] acuity & gross fields intact	Oropharynx	[] nl teeth, tongue, pharynx	Abnormals:	
Abnormals:		Abnormals:			

GI Palpation	[] no masses or tenderness [] no hep/splenomegaly	**Resp** Effort	[] nl w/o retractions	**Skin**	[] no rashes, or lesions
Ausculation	[] nl bowel sounds	Percussion	[] no dullness	Chest	[] nl breast, no d/c
Percussion	[] no dullness	Palpation	[] no fremitus	Lymph nodes	[] no axillary, inguinal, cervical or submandibular LAD
Anus/rectum	[] no abnormality or masses [] heme negative stool	Ausculation	[] CTA w/o W, R, or R	GU	[] nl male/female exam
Abnormals:		Abnormals:		Psych	[] nl cognition

CV Palpation	[] PMI nondisplaced	**Neuro** Orientation	[] AAO x 3	Abnormals:
Auscultation	[] no murmur, gallop, or rub	Cranial nerves	[] CN II-XII intact	
Carotids	[] nl intensity w/o bruit	Sensory	[] nl sensation	
JVD	[] no jugulovenous distention	Reflexes	[] 2+ & symmetrical	
Pulses	[] 2+/= femoral & pedal pulses	Abnormals:		
Edema	[] no pedal edema			
Abnormals				

Musculoskeletal	Inspection	ROM	Strength	Tone	(✓ if normal)	Abnormals:	**Other:**
Upper extremity	[]	[]	[]	[]			
Lower extremity	[]	[]	[]	[]			
Gait	[] nl gait and FROM						

Labs:

Assessment & Plan:

Clinical Rotation_____   Date: _____

Chief Complaint:
_____

History of Present Illness:
_____
_____
_____
_____
_____

Review of Systems:

	Yes	No		Yes	No		Yes	No		Yes	No
General: fatigue	[]	[]	CV: chest pain	[]	[]	Bloody stool	[]	[]	Polydypsia	[]	[]
Weight loss	[]	[]	Edema	[]	[]	GU: dysuria	[]	[]	Polyphagia	[]	[]
Fever	[]	[]	PND	[]	[]	Frequency	[]	[]	Polyphagia	[]	[]
Chills	[]	[]	Orthopnea	[]	[]	Hematuria	[]	[]	Temp int	[]	[]
Night sweats	[]	[]	Palpitations	[]	[]	Discharge	[]	[]	Derm: rash	[]	[]
Eye: vision change	[]	[]	Claudication	[]	[]	Flank pain	[]	[]	Pruritis	[]	[]
Pain	[]	[]	Resp: cough	[]	[]	MS: arthralgia	[]	[]	Neuro: weakness	[]	[]
Redness	[]	[]	SOB	[]	[]	Arthritis	[]	[]	Seizures	[]	[]
ENT: headaches	[]	[]	Wheezing	[]	[]	Joint swelling	[]	[]	Parasthesias	[]	[]
Hoarseness	[]	[]	Hemoptysis	[]	[]	Myalgias	[]	[]	Tremors	[]	[]
Sore throat	[]	[]	GI: abd pain	[]	[]	Back pain	[]	[]	Syncope	[]	[]
Epistaxis	[]	[]	BM changes	[]	[]	Heme: bleeding	[]	[]	Psych: anxiety	[]	[]
Sinus Sx	[]	[]	N/V	[]	[]	Bruising	[]	[]	Depression	[]	[]
Hearing loss	[]	[]	Diarrhea	[]	[]	Lymph: swelling	[]	[]	Hallucinations	[]	[]
Tinnitus	[]	[]	Heartburn	[]	[]	Endo: polyuria	[]	[]	All/Imm: hayfever	[]	[]
									Runny nose	[]	[]

Other ROS: _____

Past Medical History:
_____
_____
_____
_____
_____
_____

Past Surgical History:
_____
_____
_____
_____

Family History:
_____
_____

[] All other ROS reviewed and were NEGATIVE

Social History:
_____

Cigs: [] No Yes [] → Pack yrs _____
ETOH [] No Yes [] → Amount? _____
Illicits [] No Yes [] → Type? _____
Allergies: [] NKDA _____
Medications:
_____
_____
_____
_____
_____
_____
_____
_____
_____

Physical Exam   T _____   BP _____   HR _____   Wt _____(lbs)   Ht _____(in)   BMI _____

Physical Exam   T _____   BP _____   HR _____   Wt _____(lbs)   Ht _____(in)   BMI _____

Eyes	[] nl conjunctiva & lids	ENT External	[] no scars, lesions, masses	Neck External	[] no tracheal deviation
Pupils	[] equal, round, & reactive	Otoscopic	[] nl canals, TM	Palpation	[] no masses
Fundus	[] nl discs and vessels	Hearing	[] nl hearing	Thyroid	[] no enlargement
Vision	[] acuity & gross fields intact	Oropharynx	[] nl teeth, tongue, pharynx	Abnormals:	
Abnormals:		Abnormals:			

GI Palpation [] no masses or tenderness	Resp Effort [] nl w/o retractions	Skin [] no rashes, or lesions
[] no hep/splenomegaly	Percussion [] no dullness	Chest [] nl breast, no d/c
Ausculation [] nl bowel sounds	Palpation [] no fremitus	Lymph nodes [] no axillary, inguinal, cervical or submandibular LAD
Percussion [] no dullness	Ausculation [] CTA w/o W, R, or R	GU [] nl male/female exam
Anus/rectum [] no abnormality or masses [] heme negative stool	Abnormals:	Psych [] nl cognition
Abnormals:		Abnormals:

CV Palpation [] PMI nondisplaced	Neuro Orientation [] AAO x 3	
Auscultation [] no murmur, gallop, or rub	Cranial nerves [] CN II-XII intact	
Carotids [] nl intensity w/o bruit	Sensory [] nl sensation	
JVD [] no jugulovenous distention	Reflexes [] 2+ & symmetrical	
Pulses [] 2+/= femoral & pedal pulses	Abnormals:	
Edema [] no pedal edema		
Abnormals		

Musculoskeletal Inspection ROM Strength Tone (✓ if normal) Abnormals:	Other:
Upper extremity [] [] [] []	
Lower extremity [] [] [] []	
Gait [] nl gait and FROM	

Labs:

Assessment & Plan:

Clinical Rotation_____   Date: _____

Chief Complaint:
_____

History of Present Illness:
_____
_____
_____
_____
_____
_____

Review of Systems:

	Yes No		Yes No		Yes No		Yes No
General: fatigue	[] []	CV: chest pain	[] []	Bloody stool	[] []	Polydypsia	[] []
Weight loss	[] []	Edema	[] []	GU: dysuria	[] []	Polyphagia	[] []
Fever	[] []	PND	[] []	Frequency	[] []	Polyphagia	[] []
Chills	[] []	Orthopnea	[] []	Hematuria	[] []	Temp int	[] []
Night sweats	[] []	Palpitations	[] []	Discharge	[] []	Derm: rash	[] []
Eye: vision change	[] []	Claudication	[] []	Flank pain	[] []	Pruritis	[] []
Pain	[] []	Resp: cough	[] []	MS: arthralgia	[] []	Neuro: weakness	[] []
Redness	[] []	SOB	[] []	Arthritis	[] []	Seizures	[] []
ENT: headaches	[] []	Wheezing	[] []	Joint swelling	[] []	Parasthesias	[] []
Hoarseness	[] []	Hemoptysis	[] []	Myalgias	[] []	Tremors	[] []
Sore throat	[] []	GI: abd pain	[] []	Back pain	[] []	Syncope	[] []
Epistaxis	[] []	BM changes	[] []	Heme: bleeding	[] []	Psych: anxiety	[] []
Sinus Sx	[] []	N/V	[] []	Bruising	[] []	Depression	[] []
Hearing loss	[] []	Diarrhea	[] []	Lymph: swelling	[] []	Hallucinations	[] []
Tinnitus	[] []	Heartburn	[] []	Endo: polyuria	[] []	All/Imm: hayfever	[] []
						Runny nose	[] []

Other ROS: _____

Past Medical History:
_____
_____
_____
_____
_____
_____

Past Surgical History:
_____
_____
_____
_____

Family History:
_____
_____

[] All other ROS reviewed and were NEGATIVE

Social History:
_____

Cigs: [] No Yes [] → Pack yrs _____
ETOH [] No Yes [] → Amount? _____
Illicits [] No Yes [] → Type? _____
Allergies: [] NKDA _____
Medications:
_____
_____
_____
_____
_____
_____
_____
_____
_____
_____

Physical Exam T _____ BP _____ HR _____ Wt _____(lbs) Ht _____(in) BMI _____		
Eyes [] nl conjunctiva & lids	**ENT** External [] no scars, lesions, masses	**Neck** External [] no tracheal deviation
Pupils [] equal, round, & reactive	Otoscopic [] nl canals, TM	Palpation [] no masses
Fundus [] nl discs and vessels	Hearing [] nl hearing	Thyroid [] no enlargement
Vision [] acuity & gross fields intact	Oropharynx [] nl teeth, tongue, pharynx	Abnormals:
Abnormals:	Abnormals:	
GI Palpation [] no masses or tenderness [] no hep/splenomegaly	**Resp** Effort [] nl w/o retractions	**Skin** [] no rashes, or lesions
	Percussion [] no dullness	Chest [] nl breast, no d/c
Ausculation [] nl bowel sounds	Palpation [] no fremitus	Lymph nodes [] no axillary, inguinal, cervical or submandibular LAD
Percussion [] no dullness	Ausculation [] CTA w/o W, R, or R	
Anus/rectum [] no abnormality or masses [] heme negative stool	Abnormals:	GU [] nl male/female exam
Abnormals:		Psych [] nl cognition
CV Palpation [] PMI nondisplaced	**Neuro** Orientation [] AAO x 3	Abnormals:
Auscultation [] no murmur, gallop, or rub	Cranial nerves [] CN II-XII intact	
Carotids [] nl intensity w/o bruit	Sensory [] nl sensation	
JVD [] no jugulovenous distention	Reflexes [] 2+ & symmetrical	
Pulses [] 2+/= femoral & pedal pulses	Abnormals:	
Edema [] no pedal edema		
Abnormals		

Musculoskeletal Inspection ROM Strength Tone (✓ if normal) Abnormals:	**Other:**
Upper extremity [] [] [] []	
Lower extremity [] [] [] []	
Gait [] nl gait and FROM	

Labs:

Assessment & Plan:

_____
_____
_____
_____
_____
_____
_____
_____
_____
_____
_____

Clinical Rotation_____   Date: _____

Chief Complaint:
_____

History of Present Illness:
_____
_____
_____
_____
_____

Review of Systems:

	Yes	No		Yes	No		Yes	No		Yes	No
General: fatigue	[]	[]	CV: chest pain	[]	[]	Bloody stool	[]	[]	Polydypsia	[]	[]
Weight loss	[]	[]	Edema	[]	[]	GU: dysuria	[]	[]	Polyphagia	[]	[]
Fever	[]	[]	PND	[]	[]	Frequency	[]	[]	Polyphagia	[]	[]
Chills	[]	[]	Orthopnea	[]	[]	Hematuria	[]	[]	Temp int	[]	[]
Night sweats	[]	[]	Palpitations	[]	[]	Discharge	[]	[]	Derm: rash	[]	[]
Eye: vision change	[]	[]	Claudication	[]	[]	Flank pain	[]	[]	Pruritis	[]	[]
Pain	[]	[]	Resp: cough	[]	[]	MS: arthralgia	[]	[]	Neuro: weakness	[]	[]
Redness	[]	[]	SOB	[]	[]	Arthritis	[]	[]	Seizures	[]	[]
ENT: headaches	[]	[]	Wheezing	[]	[]	Joint swelling	[]	[]	Parasthesias	[]	[]
Hoarseness	[]	[]	Hemoptysis	[]	[]	Myalgias	[]	[]	Tremors	[]	[]
Sore throat	[]	[]	GI: abd pain	[]	[]	Back pain	[]	[]	Syncope	[]	[]
Epistaxis	[]	[]	BM changes	[]	[]	Heme: bleeding	[]	[]	Psych: anxiety	[]	[]
Sinus Sx	[]	[]	N/V	[]	[]	Bruising	[]	[]	Depression	[]	[]
Hearing loss	[]	[]	Diarrhea	[]	[]	Lymph: swelling	[]	[]	Hallucinations	[]	[]
Tinnitus	[]	[]	Heartburn	[]	[]	Endo: polyuria	[]	[]	All/Imm: hayfever	[]	[]
									Runny nose	[]	[]

Other ROS: _____

Past Medical History:
_____
_____
_____
_____
_____

Social History:
_____

Cigs: [] No Yes [] → Pack yrs _____
ETOH [] No Yes [] → Amount? _____
Illicits [] No Yes [] → Type?   _____
Allergies: [] NKDA _____
Medications:
_____
_____

Past Surgical History:
_____
_____
_____
_____

Family History:
_____
_____
_____
_____

[ ] All other ROS reviewed and were NEGATIVE

Physical Exam T _____ BP _____ HR _____ Wt _____ (lbs) Ht _____ (in) BMI _____		
Eyes [] nl conjunctiva & lids	**ENT** External [] no scars, lesions, masses	**Neck** External [] no tracheal deviation
Pupils [] equal, round, & reactive	Otoscopic [] nl canals, TM	Palpation [] no masses
Fundus [] nl discs and vessels	Hearing [] nl hearing	Thyroid [] no enlargement
Vision [] acuity & gross fields intact	Oropharynx [] nl teeth, tongue, pharynx	Abnormals:
Abnormals:	Abnormals:	
GI Palpation [] no masses or tenderness [] no hep/splenomegaly	**Resp** Effort [] nl w/o retractions	**Skin** [] no rashes, or lesions
Ausculation [] nl bowel sounds	Percussion [] no dullness	Chest [] nl breast, no d/c
Percussion [] no dullness	Palpation [] no fremitus	Lymph nodes [] no axillary, inguinal, cervical or submandibular LAD
Anus/rectum [] no abnormality or masses [] heme negative stool	Ausculation [] CTA w/o W, R, or R	GU [] nl male/female exam
	Abnormals:	
Abnormals:		Psych [] nl cognition
CV Palpation [] PMI nondisplaced	**Neuro** Orientation [] AAO x 3	Abnormals:
Auscultation [] no murmur, gallop, or rub	Cranial nerves [] CN II-XII intact	
Carotids [] nl intensity w/o bruit	Sensory [] nl sensation	
JVD [] no jugulovenous distention	Reflexes [] 2+ & symmetrical	
Pulses [] 2+/= femoral & pedal pulses	Abnormals:	
Edema [] no pedal edema		
Abnormals		
Musculoskeletal Inspection ROM Strength Tone (✓ if normal) Abnormals:		**Other:**
Upper extremity [] [] [] [] Lower extremity [] [] [] []		
Gait [] nl gait and FROM		

Labs:

Assessment & Plan:

_____
_____
_____
_____
_____
_____
_____
_____
_____
_____
_____
_____

Clinical Rotation_____   Date: _____

Chief Complaint:
_____

History of Present Illness:
_____
_____
_____
_____
_____

Review of Systems:

	Yes	No		Yes	No		Yes	No		Yes	No
General: fatigue	[]	[]	CV: chest pain	[]	[]	Bloody stool	[]	[]	Polydypsia	[]	[]
Weight loss	[]	[]	Edema	[]	[]	GU: dysuria	[]	[]	Polyphagia	[]	[]
Fever	[]	[]	PND	[]	[]	Frequency	[]	[]	Polyphagia	[]	[]
Chills	[]	[]	Orthopnea	[]	[]	Hematuria	[]	[]	Temp int	[]	[]
Night sweats	[]	[]	Palpitations	[]	[]	Discharge	[]	[]	Derm: rash	[]	[]
Eye: vision change	[]	[]	Claudication	[]	[]	Flank pain	[]	[]	Pruritis	[]	[]
Pain	[]	[]	Resp: cough	[]	[]	MS: arthralgia	[]	[]	Neuro: weakness	[]	[]
Redness	[]	[]	SOB	[]	[]	Arthritis	[]	[]	Seizures	[]	[]
ENT: headaches	[]	[]	Wheezing	[]	[]	Joint swelling	[]	[]	Parasthesias	[]	[]
Hoarseness	[]	[]	Hemoptysis	[]	[]	Myalgias	[]	[]	Tremors	[]	[]
Sore throat	[]	[]	GI: abd pain	[]	[]	Back pain	[]	[]	Syncope	[]	[]
Epistaxis	[]	[]	BM changes	[]	[]	Heme: bleeding	[]	[]	Psych: anxiety	[]	[]
Sinus Sx	[]	[]	N/V	[]	[]	Bruising	[]	[]	Depression	[]	[]
Hearing loss	[]	[]	Diarrhea	[]	[]	Lymph: swelling	[]	[]	Hallucinations	[]	[]
Tinnitus	[]	[]	Heartburn	[]	[]	Endo: polyuria	[]	[]	All/Imm: hayfever	[]	[]
									Runny nose	[]	[]

Other ROS: _____

Past Medical History:
_____
_____
_____
_____
_____
_____
_____

Past Surgical History:
_____
_____
_____
_____

Family History:
_____
_____
_____

[] All other ROS reviewed and were NEGATIVE

Social History:
_____

Cigs: [] No Yes [] → Pack yrs _____
ETOH [] No Yes [] → Amount? _____
Illicits [] No Yes [] → Type? _____
Allergies: [] NKDA _____
Medications:
_____
_____
_____
_____
_____
_____
_____
_____
_____
_____
_____

Physical Exam   T _____   BP _____   HR _____   Wt _____(lbs)   Ht _____(in)   BMI _____

Eyes [] nl conjunctiva & lids	**ENT** External [] no scars, lesions, masses	**Neck** External [] no tracheal deviation
Pupils [] equal, round, & reactive	Otoscopic [] nl canals, TM	Palpation [] no masses
Fundus [] nl discs and vessels	Hearing [] nl hearing	Thyroid [] no enlargement
Vision [] acuity & gross fields intact	Oropharynx [] nl teeth, tongue, pharynx	Abnormals:
Abnormals:	Abnormals:	

GI Palpation [] no masses or tenderness [] no hep/splenomegaly	**Resp** Effort [] nl w/o retractions	**Skin** [] no rashes, or lesions
Ausculation [] nl bowel sounds	Percussion [] no dullness	Chest [] nl breast, no d/c
Percussion [] no dullness	Palpation [] no fremitus	Lymph nodes [] no axillary, inguinal, cervical or submandibular LAD
Anus/rectum [] no abnormality or masses [] heme negative stool	Ausculation [] CTA w/o W, R, or R	GU [] nl male/female exam
Abnormals:	Abnormals:	Psych [] nl cognition
CV Palpation [] PMI nondisplaced	**Neuro** Orientation [] AAO x 3	Abnormals:
Auscultation [] no murmur, gallop, or rub	Cranial nerves [] CN II-XII intact	
Carotids [] nl intensity w/o bruit	Sensory [] nl sensation	
JVD [] no jugulovenous distention	Reflexes [] 2+ & symmetrical	
Pulses [] 2+/= femoral & pedal pulses	Abnormals:	
Edema [] no pedal edema		
Abnormals		

Musculoskeletal Inspection ROM Strength Tone (✓ if normal) Abnormals:	**Other:**
Upper extremity [] [] [] [] Lower extremity [] [] [] []	
Gait [] nl gait and FROM	

Labs:

Assessment & Plan:

Clinical Rotation_____   Date: _____

Chief Complaint:
_____

History of Present Illness:
_____
_____
_____
_____
_____

Review of Systems:

	Yes No		Yes No		Yes No		Yes No
General: fatigue	☐ ☐	CV: chest pain	☐ ☐	Bloody stool	☐ ☐	Polydypsia	☐ ☐
Weight loss	☐ ☐	Edema	☐ ☐	GU: dysuria	☐ ☐	Polyphagia	☐ ☐
Fever	☐ ☐	PND	☐ ☐	Frequency	☐ ☐	Polyphagia	☐ ☐
Chills	☐ ☐	Orthopnea	☐ ☐	Hematuria	☐ ☐	Temp int	☐ ☐
Night sweats	☐ ☐	Palpitations	☐ ☐	Discharge	☐ ☐	Derm: rash	☐ ☐
Eye: vision change	☐ ☐	Claudication	☐ ☐	Flank pain	☐ ☐	Pruritis	☐ ☐
Pain	☐ ☐	Resp: cough	☐ ☐	MS: arthralgia	☐ ☐	Neuro: weakness	☐ ☐
Redness	☐ ☐	SOB	☐ ☐	Arthritis	☐ ☐	Seizures	☐ ☐
ENT: headaches	☐ ☐	Wheezing	☐ ☐	Joint swelling	☐ ☐	Parasthesias	☐ ☐
Hoarseness	☐ ☐	Hemoptysis	☐ ☐	Myalgias	☐ ☐	Tremors	☐ ☐
Sore throat	☐ ☐	GI: abd pain	☐ ☐	Back pain	☐ ☐	Syncope	☐ ☐
Epistaxis	☐ ☐	BM changes	☐ ☐	Heme: bleeding	☐ ☐	Psych: anxiety	☐ ☐
Sinus Sx	☐ ☐	N/V	☐ ☐	Bruising	☐ ☐	Depression	☐ ☐
Hearing loss	☐ ☐	Diarrhea	☐ ☐	Lymph: swelling	☐ ☐	Hallucinations	☐ ☐
Tinnitus	☐ ☐	Heartburn	☐ ☐	Endo: polyuria	☐ ☐	All/Imm: hayfever	☐ ☐
						Runny nose	☐ ☐

Other ROS: _____

Past Medical History:
_____
_____
_____
_____
_____
_____

Past Surgical History:
_____
_____
_____
_____

Family History:
_____
_____
_____

Social History:
_____

Cigs: ☐ No Yes ☐ → Pack yrs _____
ETOH ☐ No Yes ☐ → Amount? _____
Illicits ☐ No Yes ☐ → Type? _____
Allergies: ☐ NKDA _____
Medications:
_____
_____
_____
_____
_____
_____
_____
_____

[] All other ROS reviewed and were NEGATIVE

Physical Exam	T _____	BP _____	HR _____	Wt _____(lbs)	Ht _____(in)	BMI _____

Eyes		**ENT** External		**Neck** External	
Eyes	[] nl conjunctiva & lids	ENT External	[] no scars, lesions, masses	Neck External	[] no tracheal deviation
Pupils	[] equal, round, & reactive	Otoscopic	[] nl canals, TM	Palpation	[] no masses
Fundus	[] nl discs and vessels	Hearing	[] nl hearing	Thyroid	[] no enlargement
Vision	[] acuity & gross fields intact	Oropharynx	[] nl teeth, tongue, pharynx	Abnormals:	
Abnormals:		Abnormals:			

GI Palpation	[] no masses or tenderness [] no hep/splenomegaly	**Resp** Effort	[] nl w/o retractions	**Skin**	[] no rashes, or lesions
Ausculation	[] nl bowel sounds	Percussion	[] no dullness	Chest	[] nl breast, no d/c
Percussion	[] no dullness	Palpation	[] no fremitus	Lymph nodes	[] no axillary, inguinal, cervical or submandibular LAD
Anus/rectum	[] no abnormality or masses [] heme negative stool	Ausculation	[] CTA w/o W, R, or R	GU	[] nl male/female exam
Abnormals:		Abnormals:		Psych	[] nl cognition

CV Palpation	[] PMI nondisplaced	**Neuro** Orientation	[] AAO x 3	Abnormals:	
Auscultation	[] no murmur, gallop, or rub	Cranial nerves	[] CN II-XII intact		
Carotids	[] nl intensity w/o bruit	Sensory	[] nl sensation		
JVD	[] no jugulovenous distention	Reflexes	[] 2+ & symmetrical		
Pulses	[] 2+/= femoral & pedal pulses	Abnormals:			
Edema	[] no pedal edema				
Abnormals					

Musculoskeletal	Inspection	ROM	Strength	Tone (✓ if normal)	Abnormals:	**Other:**
Upper extremity	[]	[]	[]	[]		
Lower extremity	[]	[]	[]	[]		
Gait	[] nl gait and FROM					

Labs:

Assessment & Plan:

_____

Clinical Rotation_____   Date: _____

Chief Complaint:

_____

History of Present Illness:

_____
_____
_____
_____
_____

Review of Systems:

	Yes	No		Yes	No		Yes	No		Yes	No
General: fatigue	[]	[]	CV: chest pain	[]	[]	Bloody stool	[]	[]	Polydypsia	[]	[]
Weight loss	[]	[]	Edema	[]	[]	GU: dysuria	[]	[]	Polyphagia	[]	[]
Fever	[]	[]	PND	[]	[]	Frequency	[]	[]	Polyphagia	[]	[]
Chills	[]	[]	Orthopnea	[]	[]	Hematuria	[]	[]	Temp int	[]	[]
Night sweats	[]	[]	Palpitations	[]	[]	Discharge	[]	[]	Derm: rash	[]	[]
Eye: vision change	[]	[]	Claudication	[]	[]	Flank pain	[]	[]	Pruritis	[]	[]
Pain	[]	[]	Resp: cough	[]	[]	MS: arthralgia	[]	[]	Neuro: weakness	[]	[]
Redness	[]	[]	SOB	[]	[]	Arthritis	[]	[]	Seizures	[]	[]
ENT: headaches	[]	[]	Wheezing	[]	[]	Joint swelling	[]	[]	Parasthesias	[]	[]
Hoarseness	[]	[]	Hemoptysis	[]	[]	Myalgias	[]	[]	Tremors	[]	[]
Sore throat	[]	[]	GI: abd pain	[]	[]	Back pain	[]	[]	Syncope	[]	[]
Epistaxis	[]	[]	BM changes	[]	[]	Heme: bleeding	[]	[]	Psych: anxiety	[]	[]
Sinus Sx	[]	[]	N/V	[]	[]	Bruising	[]	[]	Depression	[]	[]
Hearing loss	[]	[]	Diarrhea	[]	[]	Lymph: swelling	[]	[]	Hallucinations	[]	[]
Tinnitus	[]	[]	Heartburn	[]	[]	Endo: polyuria	[]	[]	All/Imm: hayfever	[]	[]
									Runny nose	[]	[]

Other ROS: _____

Past Medical History:

_____
_____
_____
_____
_____
_____

Past Surgical History:

_____
_____
_____
_____

Family History:

_____
_____
_____

[] All other ROS reviewed and were NEGATIVE

Social History:

_____

Cigs: [] No Yes [] → Pack yrs _____
ETOH [] No Yes [] → Amount? _____
Illicits [] No Yes [] → Type? _____
Allergies: [] NKDA _____
Medications:

_____
_____
_____
_____
_____
_____
_____

Physical Exam T _____ BP _____ HR _____ Wt _____(lbs) Ht _____(in) BMI _____		
Eyes [] nl conjunctiva & lids	**ENT** External [] no scars, lesions, masses	**Neck** External [] no tracheal deviation
Pupils [] equal, round, & reactive	Otoscopic [] nl canals, TM	Palpation [] no masses
Fundus [] nl discs and vessels	Hearing [] nl hearing	Thyroid [] no enlargement
Vision [] acuity & gross fields intact	Oropharynx [] nl teeth, tongue, pharynx	Abnormals:
Abnormals:	Abnormals:	
GI Palpation [] no masses or tenderness [] no hep/splenomegaly	**Resp** Effort [] nl w/o retractions	**Skin** [] no rashes, or lesions
Ausculation [] nl bowel sounds	Percussion [] no dullness	Chest [] nl breast, no d/c
Percussion [] no dullness	Palpation [] no fremitus	Lymph nodes [] no axillary, inguinal, cervical or submandibular LAD
Anus/rectum [] no abnormality or masses [] heme negative stool	Ausculation [] CTA w/o W, R, or R	GU [] nl male/female exam
Abnormals:	Abnormals:	Psych [] nl cognition
CV Palpation [] PMI nondisplaced	**Neuro** Orientation [] AAO x 3	Abnormals:
Auscultation [] no murmur, gallop, or rub	Cranial nerves [] CN II-XII intact	
Carotids [] nl intensity w/o bruit	Sensory [] nl sensation	
JVD [] no jugulovenous distention	Reflexes [] 2+ & symmetrical	
Pulses [] 2+/= femoral & pedal pulses	Abnormals:	
Edema [] no pedal edema		
Abnormals		
Musculoskeletal Inspection ROM Strength Tone (✓ if normal) Abnormals:		**Other:**
Upper extremity [] [] [] [] Lower extremity [] [] [] []		
Gait [] nl gait and FROM		

Labs:

Assessment & Plan:

_____
_____
_____
_____
_____
_____
_____
_____
_____
_____
_____

Clinical Rotation_____   Date: _____

Chief Complaint:
_____

History of Present Illness:
_____
_____
_____
_____
_____

Review of Systems:

	Yes No		Yes No		Yes No		Yes No
General: fatigue	[] []	CV: chest pain	[] []	Bloody stool	[] []	Polydypsia	[] []
Weight loss	[] []	Edema	[] []	GU: dysuria	[] []	Polyphagia	[] []
Fever	[] []	PND	[] []	Frequency	[] []	Polyphagia	[] []
Chills	[] []	Orthopnea	[] []	Hematuria	[] []	Temp int	[] []
Night sweats	[] []	Palpitations	[] []	Discharge	[] []	Derm: rash	[] []
Eye: vision change	[] []	Claudication	[] []	Flank pain	[] []	Pruritis	[] []
Pain	[] []	Resp: cough	[] []	MS: arthralgia	[] []	Neuro: weakness	[] []
Redness	[] []	SOB	[] []	Arthritis	[] []	Seizures	[] []
ENT: headaches	[] []	Wheezing	[] []	Joint swelling	[] []	Parasthesias	[] []
Hoarseness	[] []	Hemoptysis	[] []	Myalgias	[] []	Tremors	[] []
Sore throat	[] []	GI: abd pain	[] []	Back pain	[] []	Syncope	[] []
Epistaxis	[] []	BM changes	[] []	Heme: bleeding	[] []	Psych: anxiety	[] []
Sinus Sx	[] []	N/V	[] []	Bruising	[] []	Depression	[] []
Hearing loss	[] []	Diarrhea	[] []	Lymph: swelling	[] []	Hallucinations	[] []
Tinnitus	[] []	Heartburn	[] []	Endo: polyuria	[] []	All/Imm: hayfever	[] []
						Runny nose	[] []

Other ROS: _____

Past Medical History:
_____
_____
_____
_____
_____
_____
_____

Past Surgical History:
_____
_____
_____
_____

Family History:
_____
_____
_____

[] All other ROS reviewed and were NEGATIVE

Social History:
_____
_____

Cigs: [] No Yes [] → Pack yrs _____
ETOH [] No Yes [] → Amount? _____
Illicits [] No Yes [] → Type? _____
Allergies: [] NKDA _____
Medications:
_____
_____
_____
_____
_____
_____
_____
_____
_____
_____
_____
_____

Physical Exam T _____ BP _____ HR _____ Wt _____(lbs) Ht _____(in) BMI _____

Eyes [] nl conjunctiva & lids	**ENT** External [] no scars, lesions, masses	**Neck** External [] no tracheal deviation
Pupils [] equal, round, & reactive	Otoscopic [] nl canals, TM	Palpation [] no masses
Fundus [] nl discs and vessels	Hearing [] nl hearing	Thyroid [] no enlargement
Vision [] acuity & gross fields intact	Oropharynx [] nl teeth, tongue, pharynx	Abnormals:
Abnormals:	Abnormals:	
GI Palpation [] no masses or tenderness [] no hep/splenomegaly Ausculation [] nl bowel sounds Percussion [] no dullness Anus/rectum [] no abnormality or masses [] heme negative stool Abnormals:	**Resp** Effort [] nl w/o retractions Percussion [] no dullness Palpation [] no fremitus Ausculation [] CTA w/o W, R, or R Abnormals:	**Skin** [] no rashes, or lesions Chest [] nl breast, no d/c Lymph nodes [] no axillary, inguinal, cervical or submandibular LAD GU [] nl male/female exam Psych [] nl cognition
CV Palpation [] PMI nondisplaced Auscultation [] no murmur, gallop, or rub Carotids [] nl intensity w/o bruit JVD [] no jugulovenous distention Pulses [] 2+/= femoral & pedal pulses Edema [] no pedal edema Abnormals	**Neuro** Orientation [] AAO x 3 Cranial nerves [] CN II-XII intact Sensory [] nl sensation Reflexes [] 2+ & symmetrical Abnormals:	Abnormals:

Musculoskeletal Inspection ROM Strength Tone (✓ if normal) Abnormals: | **Other:**

Upper extremity [] [] [] []
Lower extremity [] [] [] []

Gait [] nl gait and FROM

Labs:

Assessment & Plan:

_____
_____
_____
_____
_____
_____
_____
_____
_____
_____
_____

Clinical Rotation_____   Date: _____

Chief Complaint:
_____

History of Present Illness:
_____
_____
_____
_____
_____

Review of Systems:

	Yes	No		Yes	No		Yes	No		Yes	No
General: fatigue	[]	[]	CV: chest pain	[]	[]	Bloody stool	[]	[]	Polydypsia	[]	[]
Weight loss	[]	[]	Edema	[]	[]	GU: dysuria	[]	[]	Polyphagia	[]	[]
Fever	[]	[]	PND	[]	[]	Frequency	[]	[]	Polyphagia	[]	[]
Chills	[]	[]	Orthopnea	[]	[]	Hematuria	[]	[]	Temp int	[]	[]
Night sweats	[]	[]	Palpitations	[]	[]	Discharge	[]	[]	Derm: rash	[]	[]
Eye: vision change	[]	[]	Claudication	[]	[]	Flank pain	[]	[]	Pruritis	[]	[]
Pain	[]	[]	Resp: cough	[]	[]	MS: arthralgia	[]	[]	Neuro: weakness	[]	[]
Redness	[]	[]	SOB	[]	[]	Arthritis	[]	[]	Seizures	[]	[]
ENT: headaches	[]	[]	Wheezing	[]	[]	Joint swelling	[]	[]	Parasthesias	[]	[]
Hoarseness	[]	[]	Hemoptysis	[]	[]	Myalgias	[]	[]	Tremors	[]	[]
Sore throat	[]	[]	GI: abd pain	[]	[]	Back pain	[]	[]	Syncope	[]	[]
Epistaxis	[]	[]	BM changes	[]	[]	Heme: bleeding	[]	[]	Psych: anxiety	[]	[]
Sinus Sx	[]	[]	N/V	[]	[]	Bruising	[]	[]	Depression	[]	[]
Hearing loss	[]	[]	Diarrhea	[]	[]	Lymph: swelling	[]	[]	Hallucinations	[]	[]
Tinnitus	[]	[]	Heartburn	[]	[]	Endo: polyuria	[]	[]	All/Imm: hayfever	[]	[]
									Runny nose	[]	[]

Other ROS:_____

Past Medical History:
_____
_____
_____
_____
_____
_____
_____

Past Surgical History:
_____
_____
_____
_____

Family History:
_____
_____

[] All other ROS reviewed and were NEGATIVE

Social History:
_____
_____

Cigs: [] No Yes [] → Pack yrs _____
ETOH [] No Yes [] → Amount? _____
Illicits [] No Yes [] → Type? _____
Allergies: [] NKDA _____
Medications:
_____
_____
_____
_____
_____
_____
_____
_____
_____
_____

Physical Exam T _____ BP _____ HR _____ Wt _____(lbs) Ht _____(in) BMI _____		
Eyes [] nl conjunctiva & lids	**ENT** External [] no scars, lesions, masses	**Neck** External [] no tracheal deviation
Pupils [] equal, round, & reactive	Otoscopic [] nl canals, TM	Palpation [] no masses
Fundus [] nl discs and vessels	Hearing [] nl hearing	Thyroid [] no enlargement
Vision [] acuity & gross fields intact	Oropharynx [] nl teeth, tongue, pharynx	Abnormals:
Abnormals:	Abnormals:	**Skin** [] no rashes, or lesions
GI Palpation [] no masses or tenderness [] no hep/splenomegaly	**Resp** Effort [] nl w/o retractions	
	Percussion [] no dullness	Chest [] nl breast, no d/c
Ausculation [] nl bowel sounds	Palpation [] no fremitus	Lymph nodes [] no axillary, inguinal, cervical or submandibular LAD
Percussion [] no dullness	Ausculation [] CTA w/o W, R, or R	
Anus/rectum [] no abnormality or masses [] heme negative stool	Abnormals:	GU [] nl male/female exam
Abnormals:		Psych [] nl cognition
CV Palpation [] PMI nondisplaced	**Neuro** Orientation [] AAO x 3	Abnormals:
Auscultation [] no murmur, gallop, or rub	Cranial nerves [] CN II-XII intact	
Carotids [] nl intensity w/o bruit	Sensory [] nl sensation	
JVD [] no jugulovenous distention	Reflexes [] 2+ & symmetrical	
Pulses [] 2+/= femoral & pedal pulses	Abnormals:	
Edema [] no pedal edema		
Abnormals		

Musculoskeletal	Inspection	ROM	Strength	Tone (✓ if normal)	Abnormals:	**Other:**
Upper extremity	[]	[]	[]	[]		
Lower extremity	[]	[]	[]	[]		
Gait	[] nl gait and FROM					

Labs:

Assessment & Plan:

_____
_____
_____
_____
_____
_____
_____
_____
_____

Clinical Rotation_____   Date: _____

Chief Complaint:
_____

History of Present Illness:
_____
_____
_____
_____
_____

Review of Systems:

	Yes	No		Yes	No		Yes	No		Yes	No
General: fatigue	[]	[]	CV: chest pain	[]	[]	Bloody stool	[]	[]	Polydypsia	[]	[]
Weight loss	[]	[]	Edema	[]	[]	GU: dysuria	[]	[]	Polyphagia	[]	[]
Fever	[]	[]	PND	[]	[]	Frequency	[]	[]	Polyphagia	[]	[]
Chills	[]	[]	Orthopnea	[]	[]	Hematuria	[]	[]	Temp int	[]	[]
Night sweats	[]	[]	Palpitations	[]	[]	Discharge	[]	[]	Derm: rash	[]	[]
Eye: vision change	[]	[]	Claudication	[]	[]	Flank pain	[]	[]	Pruritis	[]	[]
Pain	[]	[]	Resp: cough	[]	[]	MS: arthralgia	[]	[]	Neuro: weakness	[]	[]
Redness	[]	[]	SOB	[]	[]	Arthritis	[]	[]	Seizures	[]	[]
ENT: headaches	[]	[]	Wheezing	[]	[]	Joint swelling	[]	[]	Parasthesias	[]	[]
Hoarseness	[]	[]	Hemoptysis	[]	[]	Myalgias	[]	[]	Tremors	[]	[]
Sore throat	[]	[]	GI: abd pain	[]	[]	Back pain	[]	[]	Syncope	[]	[]
Epistaxis	[]	[]	BM changes	[]	[]	Heme: bleeding	[]	[]	Psych: anxiety	[]	[]
Sinus Sx	[]	[]	N/V	[]	[]	Bruising	[]	[]	Depression	[]	[]
Hearing loss	[]	[]	Diarrhea	[]	[]	Lymph: swelling	[]	[]	Hallucinations	[]	[]
Tinnitus	[]	[]	Heartburn	[]	[]	Endo: polyuria	[]	[]	All/Imm: hayfever	[]	[]
									Runny nose	[]	[]

Other ROS: _____

Past Medical History:
_____
_____
_____
_____
_____
_____

Past Surgical History:
_____
_____
_____
_____

Family History:
_____
_____

Social History:
_____

Cigs: [] No Yes [] → Pack yrs _____
ETOH [] No Yes [] → Amount? _____
Illicits [] No Yes [] → Type? _____
Allergies: [] NKDA _____
Medications:
_____
_____
_____
_____
_____
_____
_____
_____
_____
_____
_____

[] All other ROS reviewed and were NEGATIVE

Physical Exam T _____ BP _____ HR _____ Wt _____ (lbs) Ht _____ (in) BMI _____

Eyes	[] nl conjunctiva & lids	ENT External	[] no scars, lesions, masses	Neck External	[] no tracheal deviation
Pupils	[] equal, round, & reactive	Otoscopic	[] nl canals, TM	Palpation	[] no masses
Fundus	[] nl discs and vessels	Hearing	[] nl hearing	Thyroid	[] no enlargement
Vision	[] acuity & gross fields intact	Oropharynx	[] nl teeth, tongue, pharynx	Abnormals:	
Abnormals:		Abnormals:			

GI Palpation []	no masses or tenderness	Resp Effort	[] nl w/o retractions	Skin	[] no rashes, or lesions
[]	no hep/splenomegaly	Percussion	[] no dullness	Chest	[] nl breast, no d/c
Ausculation []	nl bowel sounds	Palpation	[] no fremitus	Lymph nodes []	no axillary, inguinal, cervical or submandibular LAD
Percussion []	no dullness	Ausculation	[] CTA w/o W, R, or R		
Anus/rectum []	no abnormality or masses	Abnormals:		GU	[] nl male/female exam
[]	heme negative stool			Psych	[] nl cognition
Abnormals:					

CV Palpation []	PMI nondisplaced	Neuro Orientation [] AAO x 3	Skin Abnormals:
Auscultation []	no murmur, gallop, or rub	Cranial nerves [] CN II-XII intact	
Carotids []	nl intensity w/o bruit	Sensory [] nl sensation	
JVD []	no jugulovenous distention	Reflexes [] 2+ & symmetrical	
Pulses []	2+/= femoral & pedal pulses	Abnormals:	
Edema []	no pedal edema		
Abnormals			

Musculoskeletal	Inspection	ROM	Strength	Tone (✓ if normal)	Abnormals:	Other:
Upper extremity	[]	[]	[]	[]		
Lower extremity	[]	[]	[]	[]		
Gait	[]	nl gait and FROM				

Labs:

Assessment & Plan:

_____
_____
_____
_____
_____
_____
_____
_____
_____
_____
_____

Clinical Rotation_____   Date: _____

Chief Complaint:
_____

History of Present Illness:
_____
_____
_____
_____
_____
_____

Review of Systems:

	Yes	No		Yes	No		Yes	No		Yes	No
General: fatigue	[]	[]	CV: chest pain	[]	[]	Bloody stool	[]	[]	Polydypsia	[]	[]
Weight loss	[]	[]	Edema	[]	[]	GU: dysuria	[]	[]	Polyphagia	[]	[]
Fever	[]	[]	PND	[]	[]	Frequency	[]	[]	Polyphagia	[]	[]
Chills	[]	[]	Orthopnea	[]	[]	Hematuria	[]	[]	Temp int	[]	[]
Night sweats	[]	[]	Palpitations	[]	[]	Discharge	[]	[]	Derm: rash	[]	[]
Eye: vision change	[]	[]	Claudication	[]	[]	Flank pain	[]	[]	Pruritis	[]	[]
Pain	[]	[]	Resp: cough	[]	[]	MS: arthralgia	[]	[]	Neuro: weakness	[]	[]
Redness	[]	[]	SOB	[]	[]	Arthritis	[]	[]	Seizures	[]	[]
ENT: headaches	[]	[]	Wheezing	[]	[]	Joint swelling	[]	[]	Parasthesias	[]	[]
Hoarseness	[]	[]	Hemoptysis	[]	[]	Myalgias	[]	[]	Tremors	[]	[]
Sore throat	[]	[]	GI: abd pain	[]	[]	Back pain	[]	[]	Syncope	[]	[]
Epistaxis	[]	[]	BM changes	[]	[]	Heme: bleeding	[]	[]	Psych: anxiety	[]	[]
Sinus Sx	[]	[]	N/V	[]	[]	Bruising	[]	[]	Depression	[]	[]
Hearing loss	[]	[]	Diarrhea	[]	[]	Lymph: swelling	[]	[]	Hallucinations	[]	[]
Tinnitus	[]	[]	Heartburn	[]	[]	Endo: polyuria	[]	[]	All/Imm: hayfever	[]	[]
									Runny nose	[]	[]

Other ROS: _____

Past Medical History:
_____
_____
_____
_____
_____
_____

Past Surgical History:
_____
_____
_____
_____

Family History:
_____
_____
_____

[] All other ROS reviewed and were NEGATIVE

Social History:
_____

Cigs: [] No Yes [] → Pack yrs _____
ETOH [] No Yes [] → Amount? _____
Illicits [] No Yes [] → Type? _____
Allergies: [] NKDA _____
Medications:
_____
_____
_____
_____
_____
_____
_____
_____
_____

Physical Exam T _____ BP _____ HR _____ Wt _____(lbs) Ht _____(in) BMI _____

Eyes	[] nl conjunctiva & lids	ENT External	[] no scars, lesions, masses	Neck External	[] no tracheal deviation
Pupils	[] equal, round, & reactive	Otoscopic	[] nl canals, TM	Palpation	[] no masses
Fundus	[] nl discs and vessels	Hearing	[] nl hearing	Thyroid	[] no enlargement
Vision	[] acuity & gross fields intact	Oropharynx	[] nl teeth, tongue, pharynx	Abnormals:	
Abnormals:		Abnormals:			

GI Palpation []	no masses or tenderness	Resp Effort []	nl w/o retractions	Skin	[] no rashes, or lesions
	[] no hep/splenomegaly	Percussion []	no dullness	Chest	[] nl breast, no d/c
Ausculation []	nl bowel sounds	Palpation []	no fremitus	Lymph nodes	[] no axillary, inguinal, cervical or submandibular LAD
Percussion []	no dullness	Ausculation []	CTA w/o W, R, or R		
Anus/rectum []	no abnormality or masses	Abnormals:		GU	[] nl male/female exam
[]	heme negative stool				
Abnormals:				Psych	[] nl cognition

CV Palpation []	PMI nondisplaced	Neuro Orientation []	AAO x 3	Abnormals:	
Auscultation []	no murmur, gallop, or rub	Cranial nerves []	CN II-XII intact		
Carotids []	nl intensity w/o bruit	Sensory []	nl sensation		
JVD []	no jugulovenous distention	Reflexes []	2+ & symmetrical		
Pulses []	2+/= femoral & pedal pulses	Abnormals:			
Edema []	no pedal edema				
Abnormals					

Musculoskeletal	Inspection	ROM	Strength	Tone	(✓ if normal) Abnormals:	Other:
Upper extremity	[]	[]	[]	[]		
Lower extremity	[]	[]	[]	[]		
Gait	[] nl gait and FROM					

Labs:

Assessment & Plan:

_____
_____
_____
_____
_____
_____
_____
_____
_____
_____
_____

Clinical Rotation_____   Date: _____

Chief Complaint:
_____

History of Present Illness:
_____
_____
_____
_____
_____

Review of Systems:

	Yes No		Yes No		Yes No		Yes No
General: fatigue	[] []	CV: chest pain	[] []	Bloody stool	[] []	Polydypsia	[] []
Weight loss	[] []	Edema	[] []	GU: dysuria	[] []	Polyphagia	[] []
Fever	[] []	PND	[] []	Frequency	[] []	Polyphagia	[] []
Chills	[] []	Orthopnea	[] []	Hematuria	[] []	Temp int	[] []
Night sweats	[] []	Palpitations	[] []	Discharge	[] []	Derm: rash	[] []
Eye: vision change	[] []	Claudication	[] []	Flank pain	[] []	Pruritis	[] []
Pain	[] []	Resp: cough	[] []	MS: arthralgia	[] []	Neuro: weakness	[] []
Redness	[] []	SOB	[] []	Arthritis	[] []	Seizures	[] []
ENT: headaches	[] []	Wheezing	[] []	Joint swelling	[] []	Parasthesias	[] []
Hoarseness	[] []	Hemoptysis	[] []	Myalgias	[] []	Tremors	[] []
Sore throat	[] []	GI: abd pain	[] []	Back pain	[] []	Syncope	[] []
Epistaxis	[] []	BM changes	[] []	Heme: bleeding	[] []	Psych: anxiety	[] []
Sinus Sx	[] []	N/V	[] []	Bruising	[] []	Depression	[] []
Hearing loss	[] []	Diarrhea	[] []	Lymph: swelling	[] []	Hallucinations	[] []
Tinnitus	[] []	Heartburn	[] []	Endo: polyuria	[] []	All/Imm: hayfever	[] []
						Runny nose	[] []

Other ROS: _____

Past Medical History:
_____
_____
_____
_____
_____
_____

Past Surgical History:
_____
_____
_____
_____

Family History:
_____
_____

[] All other ROS reviewed and were NEGATIVE

Social History:
_____

Cigs: [] No Yes [] → Pack yrs _____
ETOH [] No Yes [] → Amount? _____
Illicits [] No Yes [] → Type? _____
Allergies: [] NKDA _____
Medications:
_____
_____
_____
_____
_____
_____
_____
_____

Physical Exam T _____ BP _____ HR _____ Wt _____(lbs) Ht _____(in) BMI _____

Eyes	[] nl conjunctiva & lids	**ENT** External	[] no scars, lesions, masses	**Neck** External	[]	no tracheal deviation
Pupils	[] equal, round, & reactive	Otoscopic	[] nl canals, TM	Palpation	[]	no masses
Fundus	[] nl discs and vessels	Hearing	[] nl hearing	Thyroid	[]	no enlargement
Vision	[] acuity & gross fields intact	Oropharynx	[] nl teeth, tongue, pharynx	Abnormals:		
Abnormals:		Abnormals:				

GI Palpation []	no masses or tenderness	**Resp** Effort	[] nl w/o retractions	**Skin**	[]	no rashes, or lesions
[]	no hep/splenomegaly	Percussion	[] no dullness	Chest	[]	nl breast, no d/c
Ausculation []	nl bowel sounds	Palpation	[] no fremitus	Lymph nodes	[]	no axillary, inguinal, cervical or submandibular LAD
Percussion []	no dullness	Ausculation	[] CTA w/o W, R, or R			
Anus/rectum []	no abnormality or masses	Abnormals:		GU	[]	nl male/female exam
[]	heme negative stool			Psych	[]	nl cognition
Abnormals:				Abnormals:		

CV Palpation []	PMI nondisplaced	**Neuro** Orientation [] AAO x 3		
Auscultation []	no murmur, gallop, or rub	Cranial nerves	[] CN II-XII intact	
Carotids []	nl intensity w/o bruit	Sensory	[] nl sensation	
JVD []	no jugulovenous distention	Reflexes	[] 2+ & symmetrical	
Pulses []	2+/= femoral & pedal pulses	Abnormals:		
Edema []	no pedal edema			
Abnormals				

Musculoskeletal	Inspection	ROM	Strength	Tone (✓ if normal)	Abnormals:	**Other:**
Upper extremity	[]	[]	[]	[]		
Lower extremity	[]	[]	[]	[]		
Gait	[] nl gait and FROM					

Labs:

Assessment & Plan:

_____
_____
_____
_____
_____
_____
_____
_____
_____
_____

Clinical Rotation_____   Date: _____

Chief Complaint:
_____

History of Present Illness:
_____
_____
_____
_____
_____
_____

Review of Systems:

	Yes	No		Yes	No		Yes	No		Yes	No
General: fatigue	[]	[]	CV: chest pain	[]	[]	Bloody stool	[]	[]	Polydypsia	[]	[]
Weight loss	[]	[]	Edema	[]	[]	GU: dysuria	[]	[]	Polyphagia	[]	[]
Fever	[]	[]	PND	[]	[]	Frequency	[]	[]	Polyphagia	[]	[]
Chills	[]	[]	Orthopnea	[]	[]	Hematuria	[]	[]	Temp int	[]	[]
Night sweats	[]	[]	Palpitations	[]	[]	Discharge	[]	[]	Derm: rash	[]	[]
Eye: vision change	[]	[]	Claudication	[]	[]	Flank pain	[]	[]	Pruritis	[]	[]
Pain	[]	[]	Resp: cough	[]	[]	MS: arthralgia	[]	[]	Neuro: weakness	[]	[]
Redness	[]	[]	SOB	[]	[]	Arthritis	[]	[]	Seizures	[]	[]
ENT: headaches	[]	[]	Wheezing	[]	[]	Joint swelling	[]	[]	Parasthesias	[]	[]
Hoarseness	[]	[]	Hemoptysis	[]	[]	Myalgias	[]	[]	Tremors	[]	[]
Sore throat	[]	[]	GI: abd pain	[]	[]	Back pain	[]	[]	Syncope	[]	[]
Epistaxis	[]	[]	BM changes	[]	[]	Heme: bleeding	[]	[]	Psych: anxiety	[]	[]
Sinus Sx	[]	[]	N/V	[]	[]	Bruising	[]	[]	Depression	[]	[]
Hearing loss	[]	[]	Diarrhea	[]	[]	Lymph: swelling	[]	[]	Hallucinations	[]	[]
Tinnitus	[]	[]	Heartburn	[]	[]	Endo: polyuria	[]	[]	All/Imm: hayfever	[]	[]
									Runny nose	[]	[]

Other ROS: _____

Past Medical History:
_____
_____
_____
_____
_____
_____

Past Surgical History:
_____
_____
_____
_____

Family History:
_____
_____

[ ] All other ROS reviewed and were NEGATIVE

Social History:
_____

Cigs: [] No Yes [] → Pack yrs _____
ETOH [] No Yes [] → Amount? _____
Illicits [] No Yes [] → Type? _____
Allergies: [] NKDA _____
Medications:
_____
_____
_____
_____
_____
_____
_____
_____
_____

| **Physical Exam** | T _____ | BP _____ | HR _____ | Wt _____(lbs) | Ht _____(in) | BMI _____ |

Eyes	[] nl conjunctiva & lids	**ENT** External	[] no scars, lesions, masses	**Neck** External	[] no tracheal deviation
Pupils	[] equal, round, & reactive	Otoscopic	[] nl canals, TM	Palpation	[] no masses
Fundus	[] nl discs and vessels	Hearing	[] nl hearing	Thyroid	[] no enlargement
Vision	[] acuity & gross fields intact	Oropharynx	[] nl teeth, tongue, pharynx	Abnormals:	
Abnormals:		Abnormals:			

GI Palpation []	no masses or tenderness	**Resp** Effort	[] nl w/o retractions	**Skin**	[] no rashes, or lesions
[]	no hep/splenomegaly	Percussion	[] no dullness	Chest	[] nl breast, no d/c
Ausculation []	nl bowel sounds	Palpation	[] no fremitus	Lymph nodes	[] no axillary, inguinal, cervical or submandibular LAD
Percussion []	no dullness	Ausculation	[] CTA w/o W, R, or R		
Anus/rectum []	no abnormality or masses	Abnormals:		GU	[] nl male/female exam
[]	heme negative stool			Psych	[] nl cognition
Abnormals:				Abnormals:	

CV Palpation []	PMI nondisplaced	**Neuro** Orientation []	AAO x 3
Auscultation []	no murmur, gallop, or rub	Cranial nerves []	CN II-XII intact
Carotids []	nl intensity w/o bruit	Sensory []	nl sensation
JVD []	no jugulovenous distention	Reflexes []	2+ & symmetrical
Pulses []	2+/= femoral & pedal pulses	Abnormals:	
Edema []	no pedal edema		
Abnormals			

Musculoskeletal	Inspection	ROM	Strength	Tone (✓ if normal)	Abnormals:	**Other:**
Upper extremity	[]	[]	[]	[]		
Lower extremity	[]	[]	[]	[]		
Gait	[] nl gait and FROM					

Labs:

Assessment & Plan:

_____
_____
_____
_____
_____
_____
_____
_____
_____
_____
_____

Clinical Rotation_____   Date: _____

Chief Complaint:

_____

History of Present Illness:

_____
_____
_____
_____
_____

Review of Systems:

	Yes No		Yes No		Yes No		Yes No
General: fatigue	[] []	CV: chest pain	[] []	Bloody stool	[] []	Polydypsia	[] []
Weight loss	[] []	Edema	[] []	GU: dysuria	[] []	Polyphagia	[] []
Fever	[] []	PND	[] []	Frequency	[] []	Polyphagia	[] []
Chills	[] []	Orthopnea	[] []	Hematuria	[] []	Temp int	[] []
Night sweats	[] []	Palpitations	[] []	Discharge	[] []	Derm: rash	[] []
Eye: vision change	[] []	Claudication	[] []	Flank pain	[] []	Pruritis	[] []
Pain	[] []	Resp: cough	[] []	MS: arthralgia	[] []	Neuro: weakness	[] []
Redness	[] []	SOB	[] []	Arthritis	[] []	Seizures	[] []
ENT: headaches	[] []	Wheezing	[] []	Joint swelling	[] []	Parasthesias	[] []
Hoarseness	[] []	Hemoptysis	[] []	Myalgias	[] []	Tremors	[] []
Sore throat	[] []	GI: abd pain	[] []	Back pain	[] []	Syncope	[] []
Epistaxis	[] []	BM changes	[] []	Heme: bleeding	[] []	Psych: anxiety	[] []
Sinus Sx	[] []	N/V	[] []	Bruising	[] []	Depression	[] []
Hearing loss	[] []	Diarrhea	[] []	Lymph: swelling	[] []	Hallucinations	[] []
Tinnitus	[] []	Heartburn	[] []	Endo: polyuria	[] []	All/Imm: hayfever	[] []
						Runny nose	[] []

Other ROS: _____

Past Medical History:

Social History:

_____

Cigs: [] No Yes [] → Pack yrs _____
ETOH [] No Yes [] → Amount? _____
Illicits [] No Yes [] → Type? _____
Allergies: [] NKDA _____
Medications:

_____
_____
_____
_____
_____
_____

Past Surgical History:

_____
_____
_____
_____

Family History:

_____
_____

[] All other ROS reviewed and were NEGATIVE

Physical Exam	T _____	BP _____	HR _____	Wt _____(lbs)	Ht _____(in)	BMI _____

Eyes	[] nl conjunctiva & lids	**ENT** External	[] no scars, lesions, masses	**Neck** External	[] no tracheal deviation
Pupils	[] equal, round, & reactive	Otoscopic	[] nl canals, TM	Palpation	[] no masses
Fundus	[] nl discs and vessels	Hearing	[] nl hearing	Thyroid	[] no enlargement
Vision	[] acuity & gross fields intact	Oropharynx	[] nl teeth, tongue, pharynx	Abnormals:	
Abnormals:		Abnormals:			

GI Palpation	[] no masses or tenderness [] no hep/splenomegaly	**Resp** Effort	[] nl w/o retractions	**Skin**	[] no rashes, or lesions
		Percussion	[] no dullness	Chest	[] nl breast, no d/c
Ausculation	[] nl bowel sounds	Palpation	[] no fremitus	Lymph nodes	[] no axillary, inguinal, cervical or submandibular LAD
Percussion	[] no dullness	Ausculation	[] CTA w/o W, R, or R		
Anus/rectum	[] no abnormality or masses [] heme negative stool	Abnormals:		GU	[] nl male/female exam
Abnormals:				Psych	[] nl cognition

CV Palpation	[] PMI nondisplaced	**Neuro** Orientation	[] AAO x 3	Abnormals:
Auscultation	[] no murmur, gallop, or rub	Cranial nerves	[] CN II-XII intact	
Carotids	[] nl intensity w/o bruit	Sensory	[] nl sensation	
JVD	[] no jugulovenous distention	Reflexes	[] 2+ & symmetrical	
Pulses	[] 2+/= femoral & pedal pulses	Abnormals:		
Edema	[] no pedal edema			
Abnormals				

Musculoskeletal	Inspection	ROM	Strength	Tone	(✓ if normal)	Abnormals:	**Other:**
Upper extremity	[]	[]	[]	[]			
Lower extremity	[]	[]	[]	[]			
Gait	[] nl gait and FROM						

Labs:

Assessment & Plan:

_____
_____
_____
_____
_____
_____
_____
_____
_____
_____
_____
_____

Clinical Rotation_____   Date: _____

Chief Complaint:
_____

History of Present Illness:
_____
_____
_____
_____
_____

Review of Systems:

	Yes	No		Yes	No		Yes	No		Yes	No
General: fatigue	[]	[]	CV: chest pain	[]	[]	Bloody stool	[]	[]	Polydypsia	[]	[]
Weight loss	[]	[]	Edema	[]	[]	GU: dysuria	[]	[]	Polyphagia	[]	[]
Fever	[]	[]	PND	[]	[]	Frequency	[]	[]	Polyphagia	[]	[]
Chills	[]	[]	Orthopnea	[]	[]	Hematuria	[]	[]	Temp int	[]	[]
Night sweats	[]	[]	Palpitations	[]	[]	Discharge	[]	[]	Derm: rash	[]	[]
Eye: vision change	[]	[]	Claudication	[]	[]	Flank pain	[]	[]	Pruritis	[]	[]
Pain	[]	[]	Resp: cough	[]	[]	MS: arthralgia	[]	[]	Neuro: weakness	[]	[]
Redness	[]	[]	SOB	[]	[]	Arthritis	[]	[]	Seizures	[]	[]
ENT: headaches	[]	[]	Wheezing	[]	[]	Joint swelling	[]	[]	Parasthesias	[]	[]
Hoarseness	[]	[]	Hemoptysis	[]	[]	Myalgias	[]	[]	Tremors	[]	[]
Sore throat	[]	[]	GI: abd pain	[]	[]	Back pain	[]	[]	Syncope	[]	[]
Epistaxis	[]	[]	BM changes	[]	[]	Heme: bleeding	[]	[]	Psych: anxiety	[]	[]
Sinus Sx	[]	[]	N/V	[]	[]	Bruising	[]	[]	Depression	[]	[]
Hearing loss	[]	[]	Diarrhea	[]	[]	Lymph: swelling	[]	[]	Hallucinations	[]	[]
Tinnitus	[]	[]	Heartburn	[]	[]	Endo: polyuria	[]	[]	All/Imm: hayfever	[]	[]
									Runny nose	[]	[]

Other ROS: _____

Past Medical History:
_____
_____
_____
_____
_____
_____

Social History:
_____

Cigs: [] No Yes [] → Pack yrs _____
ETOH [] No Yes [] → Amount? _____
Illicits [] No Yes [] → Type? _____
Allergies: [] NKDA _____
Medications:
_____
_____

Past Surgical History:
_____
_____
_____
_____

Family History:
_____
_____
_____
_____

[] All other ROS reviewed and were NEGATIVE

Physical Exam T _____ BP _____ HR _____ Wt _____(lbs) Ht _____(in) BMI _____

Eyes			ENT			Neck		
Eyes	[]	nl conjunctiva & lids	ENT External	[]	no scars, lesions, masses	Neck External	[]	no tracheal deviation
Pupils	[]	equal, round, & reactive	Otoscopic	[]	nl canals, TM	Palpation	[]	no masses
Fundus	[]	nl discs and vessels	Hearing	[]	nl hearing	Thyroid	[]	no enlargement
Vision	[]	acuity & gross fields intact	Oropharynx	[]	nl teeth, tongue, pharynx	Abnormals:		
Abnormals:			Abnormals:					

GI Palpation	[]	no masses or tenderness	Resp Effort	[]	nl w/o retractions	Skin	[]	no rashes, or lesions
	[]	no hep/splenomegaly	Percussion	[]	no dullness	Chest	[]	nl breast, no d/c
Ausculation	[]	nl bowel sounds	Palpation	[]	no fremitus	Lymph nodes	[]	no axillary, inguinal, cervical or submandibular LAD
Percussion	[]	no dullness	Ausculation	[]	CTA w/o W, R, or R			
Anus/rectum	[]	no abnormality or masses	Abnormals:			GU	[]	nl male/female exam
	[]	heme negative stool				Psych	[]	nl cognition
Abnormals:								

CV Palpation	[]	PMI nondisplaced	Neuro Orientation	[]	AAO x 3	Abnormals:		
Auscultation	[]	no murmur, gallop, or rub	Cranial nerves	[]	CN II-XII intact			
Carotids	[]	nl intensity w/o bruit	Sensory	[]	nl sensation			
JVD	[]	no jugulovenous distention	Reflexes	[]	2+ & symmetrical			
Pulses	[]	2+/= femoral & pedal pulses	Abnormals:					
Edema	[]	no pedal edema						
Abnormals								

Musculoskeletal	Inspection	ROM	Strength	Tone (✓ if normal)	Abnormals:	Other:
Upper extremity	[]	[]	[]	[]		
Lower extremity	[]	[]	[]	[]		
Gait	[]	nl gait and FROM				

Labs:

Assessment & Plan:

Other Books by Nachole Johnson

Medical Mnemonics for the Family Nurse Practitioner

NP School and Beyond: Tips for the Student Nurse Practitioner

The Financially Savvy Nurse Practitioner: Your Guide to Building Wealth

50+ Business Ideas For The Entrepreneurial Nurse

You're a Nurse and Want to Start Your Own Business? The Complete Guide

Adult-Gero and Family Nurse Practitioner Certification Review: Labs For Primary Care

Adult-Gero and Family Nurse Practitioner Certification Review: Mental Health

Adult-Gero and Family Nurse Practitioner Certification Review: Cardiac

Adult-Gero and Family Nurse Practitioner Certification Review: Health Promotion

Adult-Gero and Family Nurse Practitioner Certification Review: Pulmonary

Adult-Gero and Family Nurse Practitioner Certification Review:

Genitourinary and STDs

Adult-Gero and Family Nurse Practitioner Certification Review: Neurology

Nachole's Amazon Author Page: amazon.com/author/nacholejohnson

Nachole's Blog: renursing.com

Notes

Notes

Made in the USA
Middletown, DE
06 January 2025